People's
Medical
Society

The Consumer's Guide to
MEDICAL
LINGO

OTHER BOOKS FROM THE PEOPLE'S MEDICAL SOCIETY

Take This Book to the Hospital With You

How to Evaluate and Select a Nursing Home

Medicine on Trial

Medicare Made Easy

Your Medical Rights

Getting the Most for Your Medical Dollar

Take This Book to the Gynecologist With You

Take This Book to the Obstetrician With You

Healthy Body Book: Test Yourself for Maximum Health

Blood Pressure: Questions You Have...Answers You Need

Your Heart: Questions You Have...Answers You Need

The Consumer's Guide to Medical Lingo

150 Ways to Be a Savvy Medical Consumer

100 Ways to Live to 100

Take This Book to the Pediatrician With You

Charles B. Inlander
President, People's Medical Society
and
Paula Brisco

The Consumer's Guide to
MEDICAL
LINGO

People's
Medical
Society
Allentown, PA

ISBN 0-9627334-4-x

CONTENTS

The Empowered Medical Consumer

The consumerism movement was born in the 1960s. Led by activists such as Ralph Nader, the movement swept through the United States with such speed and fervor that by the middle of the 1970s most states and the federal government had passed laws protecting citizens from inferior products, services, and treatment. But when it came to medical and health matters, the laws and the lawmakers remained silent. Today, while change is in the wind, medicine and health care remain the last bastions of nonconsumerism in America.

According to the federal government, health care now consumes 12 percent of the gross national product. Health care expenditures are twice that of the national defense budget. America is a medical mecca with the most sophisticated equipment and facilities in the world.

The U.S. has more doctors per capita than any other nation. While this country does not have a national health insurance program, the Medicare and Medicaid programs spend more on health care for the elderly and the poor than any other country does on its entire national health care program.

Over 36 million operations are performed in hospitals an-nually. Millions more are performed on an outpatient basis. Con-sumers undergo hundreds of millions of medical tests each year. Americans are prescribed more drugs than any other country's residents and use more than half of the world's production of pharmaceuticals annually.

Obviously, medicine in America is big business—so big that the health care industry itself is becoming the nation's largest employer. In many major metropolitan areas, health care entities are the biggest employers.

Use of the health care system is growing. Even with a signifi-cant shift away from inpatient hospital care to ambulatory ser-vices and a reduction in the average length of stay for those who are hospitalized, overall use of health care services is increas-ing. Much of this has to do with the aging of the population. Longer life brings a greater likelihood of medical encounters.

Use of the system is not limited to encounters with traditional medical entities. Aside from allopathic medical doctors (M.D.'s) and conventional hospital and ambulatory care settings, record numbers of consumers are using what some call nontraditional, alternative, or nonconventional medical services. Chiropractors, for example, are flourishing: The American Chiropractic Associa-tion claims that one out of every four Americans has seen a chiropractor. Massage therapists, acupuncturists, naturopaths, and a wide range of other medical and health professionals are seeing more patients each year. From a health care delivery standpoint, citizens have a wider range of practitioners to choose from than ever before.

Even within the traditional medical disciplines, options are greater. The number of specialists grows each year—as does the number of specialties. In 1980 few people had heard of a spe-cialty in sports medicine. Today there are practitioners who specialize in sports gynecology.

Some observers (the People's Medical Society among them) contend that the medical profession is now creating medical needs where little or no specialization is necessary. Yale School of Medicine Professor Lowell S. Levin, Ed.D., who is chair of the People's Medical Society Board of Directors, has written that the medical profession is making health itself a disease. He points out that consumers are warned not to exercise, to participate in certain activities known to improve health, or to alter what might be a poor diet without first consulting a physician. In many instances, Levin notes, physicians are no more knowledgeable about the planned activity or life-style change than their consumer customers.

There is evidence that the expansion of specialties has as much to do with a glut of practitioners as it does with medical need. In most urban areas, there are simply more practitioners than necessary. The evidence suggests that the glut will not only continue but become larger. Medical schools are spewing out physicians at a rate that far exceeds expected needs.

For the typical health care consumer, the proliferation of practitioners and specialties leads to confusion and frustration. Overspecialization results in consumers being referred from one practitioner to another for the same condition. It may mean a consumer sees one doctor for one stage of treatment and another doctor for the next stage. It may mean new jargon for the consumer to understand. In practical terms, it tends to make the final stack of bills impossible to decipher.

Pick the Facility, Pay the Bills

A proliferation of practitioners is not all that confronts the medical consumer. The settings in which health care is currently delivered are vastly different from those of the early 1980s.

At that time, most consumers received their medical care at either a doctor's office or a hospital. Today the doctor's office and hospital remain, but they have been joined by a variety of new facilities: freestanding surgical centers (surgicenters), freestanding emergency centers (emergicenters), outpatient facilities that specialize in such services as lens implantation or arthroscopic knee surgery (to name just two), plus a variety of other stand-alone service centers. Consumers can choose a private doctor, a group practice, a health maintenance organization (HMO), a preferred provider organization (PPO), or any other of a host of health care providers with acronym names.

Going to the doctor is not as simple as it was. And if these trends continue, it's not going to be any easier.

Nor is it getting easier to pay for health care. Medical inflation in the last 10 years has been three to four times that of overall inflation. Hospital and doctor fees have been rising an average of 8 to 10 percent per year. Insurance premiums in the latter part of the 1980s rose 10 to 80 percent *a year* for most payers. The nation's elderly watched as Medicare Part B premiums went up 38 percent in 1988 alone.

In October 1991 the federal government's Health Care Financing Administration reported these *out-of-pocket* health care expenses for each man, woman, and child for the year 1990:

Doctors	$112
Drugs and medical sundries	108
Nursing homes	86
Dentists	85
Hospitals	79
Chiropractors, physical therapists, and other professional services	28
Eyeglasses, contact lenses, and accessories	26

(Source: *Health Care Financing Review* [Fall 1991])

These figures *do not* include any insurance premiums. Thus, each person in America paid $524 (and a family of four over $2,000) out of pocket for health care *plus* insurance premiums.

That's a hefty price tag. Yet in 1991, 31 to 37 million Americans were without health insurance. It is estimated that over half were fully employed! The Pennsylvania Health Care Cost Containment Council, a state-created agency, released a study in 1988 showing that the uninsured were not necessarily homeless or unemployed persons. The report showed that the majority were the so-called working poor. The plight of these uninsured people was that employers could not afford to provide health insurance benefits. Nor could the employees themselves afford the premium contribution required from the weekly paycheck. Sadly, the numbers of uninsured and underinsured are growing, not declining.

Even those people with health insurance are facing higher out-of-pocket expenses. In an effort to control health care costs, companies alter their health benefits programs. Many force employees to pay a part, or larger part, of insurance premiums. They require employees to pay larger deductibles and co-payments for health services. Some companies limit benefits or eligibility to certain services. All in all, as the Health Care Financing Administration's 1990 statistics showed, 28 percent of the U.S. health care expenditure was coming from consumers' pockets.

The bottom line for the consumer is this: People must be informed and empowered to get the most from a system so vital to their well-being. This is a new phenomenon in America. Never before have the consumers of health care needed, or at least felt the need, to have as much health care and medical information as they do now.

Knowledge Is Power

Unfortunately, information about the health care system and the world of medicine is often inaccessible to consumers. Information about doctors, hospitals, and other service entities is often not in the public domain. Information about the people who provide medical care in a given community and the facilities where they work is frequently nonexistent or exempted from public disclosure. And consumer access to information about health and medical conditions, treatments, and other services related to a person's health care needs is often difficult.

Because people have traditionally not worried about health care service provision, because they historically trusted their doctor and hospital, and because the average consumer has been a passive user of medical services, the typical health care customer is not only uninformed about his or her condition but is equally in the dark as to where to look to find information.

Even the most highly educated members of our society generally lack knowledge about health and medical matters. So do the high rollers. It is not unusual for chief executive officers of major corporations to be uninformed or misinformed about their company's health insurance benefits or Medicare's provisions upon retirement. Many of our titans of industry become passive and childlike at the hands of the medical system—simply because they, like most American consumers, are ignorant about health and medical matters.

The winds of change are beginning to blow in America, as they have in Eastern Europe. Over the coming decades the U.S. is going to see the most important and biggest revolution in the history of American medicine. The medical revolutions of the past have involved drug discoveries, nutritional knowledge, medical equipment, and surgical or treatment techniques; this revolution will be the empowered consumer.

No longer will medical and health knowledge be solely in the hands of the providers. No longer will the language of medicine be a cryptic code. No longer will the treatment and care of people be in the hands of a small group of practitioners who own the machines and the journals. Informed consumers will start a series of sweeping changes, just as they did 30 years ago in areas such as automotive repair, safety, and recall disclosure; mortgage and lending disclosure; funeral disclosure requirements; and environmental issues.

Thanks to consumer effort, every state has laws that require automobile service departments to provide written estimates of work and return used parts upon customer request, and that prohibit those departments from levying charges above a cost estimate.

In banking, the consumer revolution brought about federal and state lending disclosure requirements that grant the consumer a look-see period and give customers full information about interest rates and payments.

Until recently the world of health care has been a closed, secretive society—a medical Albania. In many ways it still is. *Perestroika* has yet to materialize in matters of health and medicine.

For example, fewer than two-thirds of our states have statutes that require physicians and hospitals to give consumers copies of their medical records upon request. Most states do not require courts that have found physicians guilty of medical malpractice to report the verdict to state medical licensing boards —the only entities authorized to revoke or suspend licenses. There are no federal laws that require inserts describing contraindications and cautions in prescription medication containers dispensed to consumers.

With the exception of X-ray equipment, medical equipment generally lacks regulatory inspection for safety problems once it falls into the hands of physicians or hospitals. In fact, most states require butcher scales to be inspected at least once a year for accuracy (to protect the consumer from being ripped off), while not a single state requires physicians' blood pressure cuffs to be inspected or calibrated.

In 1989 a federal law went into effect establishing a National Practitioner Data Bank. The bank gathers information about actions that have been taken against physicians and other practitioners by hospitals, licensing boards, and courts (including settlements against the physician). The purpose of the data bank is to protect the consumer from bad practitioners who move to another state before or after disciplinary action is taken against the practitioner in the home state. Hospitals and licensing boards are required to look at the data on a prescribed basis. The theory is that by so doing they will not hire or allow bad practitioners to do business. But the law only requires that they look at the data—*it does not require that they do anything as a result of finding something.* Even more heinous is the law's provision that excludes public access to the data. Obviously, the medical industry's lobby was more powerful than consumer interests at the time the bill was passed.

But consumers are rising in response. A public outcry is growing over the failure of legislators to protect the public from the interests of the practitioners. That's the same sort of medical consumerism seen in the consumer backlash over the Catastrophic Health Care Act of 1988 and its subsequent revocation by Congress.

On a day-to-day level, consumers are demanding to know more about their health conditions and the procedures and treatments they are receiving. Letters to the editors of prestigious medical publications such as the *New England Journal of Medicine* and the *Journal of the American Medical Association* document physicians' awareness that consumers are asking more questions not only about the treatments consumers receive, but also about the training and competence of the practitioners themselves.

Because of the mounting demand for provider accountability, friction is developing between that segment of the medical profession that is reluctant to change and a citizenry that will not accept the old ways. No surprise that consumers are creating their own means of access to the information they need to make informed medical decisions. Consider these examples of a major change in the public's desire to have more information:

• In several locations across the country, consumer health libraries have emerged. The Center for Medical Consumers in New York City and the Planetree Health Resource Center in San Francisco are two of the most prominent. Both report strong consumer interest.

- In response to public demand, many hospitals have opened their in-house medical libraries to the public at certain hours.
- Bookstores do brisk business in their health sections. The nonfiction best-seller lists average one or two health books in the Top 10. Such best-selling status of health books was unheard of a decade ago.
- Consumer organizations like the People's Medical Society have emerged as strong and viable sources of consumer health information over the past decade.

What Did You Say?

One of the brick walls the medical consumer faces when trying to track down medical and health information is the medical jargon itself. The words of the trade are alien—and numerous. Doctors and pharmacists, for instance, use over 5,500 medical abbreviations. Medical dictionaries tabulate over 50,000 regularly used medical words. Consumers can look up terms in a medical dictionary, but since many of the terms are rooted in Latin or Greek, trying to understand the definition is a deeper adventure into medical confusion.

Consider the case of the consumer who has been told her spouse suffered a myocardial infarction. If she looks up the definition of *myocardial*, she'll learn it has something to do with the heart. But what should she make of this definition of *infarct*—"a necrotic area of tissue resulting from failure of local blood supply"? If the doctor had simply told her, "Your husband has had a heart attack," she would have immediately understood. If the dictionary had done the same, the problem would have been quickly solved. If a consumer-oriented glossary of medical terminology were in her home, time would have been saved.

And that's where this book comes in. Certainly, there are many consumer-oriented medical dictionaries on the market. Most are quite good, and an interested medical consumer should make use of one as needs arise. But even these dictionaries are overwhelming. Despite their alleged consumer orientation, they tend to be written for those well acquainted with the medical profession. It is not unusual for a consumer to look up half the words in a definition before getting a clue to the meaning of the original term.

This book is different. The purpose of *The Consumer's Guide to Medical Lingo* is to empower you as a medical consumer. And empowerment entails more than the opportunity to look up a word, disease, or medical condition. It is your key to taking charge of your own health management.

What is an empowered medical consumer? Simply, it is a person who either has the information necessary to make a medical decision or knows what, whom, or where to ask to become informed. In other words, it is a person who becomes as self-reliant as possible in the decision-making process of matters related to his or her own medical well-being.

Don't be misled into thinking you can do it all by yourself. You can't. Rather, the idea is to create a partnership with your health care provider. But that partnership must be an equal one, with you ultimately making the final decisions about the course of your treatment.

To be equal, you and your health care provider must speak the same language. Not much is communicated when two people do not understand the words the other utters. So it is with medicine.

In this book you'll find the most important terms you need to build the maximum partnership with your medical professionals. Use this book as a translator, similar to those in the international language business. But also use this book as a means of gaining insight into the key terms used throughout medicine.

Of course, the ideal situation would be if your doctor learned plain old ordinary English, rather than Greek- or Latin-based doctor-talk. But you cannot wait for that to occur. You must grab this book by the jacket and take control.

The changes that are occurring in medicine are dramatic. New technology and treatments have tremendous potential to enhance the lives of millions of people. But some changes are not beneficial. The days of the family doctor's house calls are gone. Today's practitioners are businesspeople, for better or for worse. They are highly trained technological marvels, skilled in technique but often lacking in human relation skills.

There are also changes in how we, as consumers, are perceived by medical practitioners. As we become more assertive, questioning, and skeptical of our medical care, we are often seen as a threat—a thorn in the professional side. Practitioners fear what we might do if they fail us. They worry about our gaining medical knowledge, concerned that we might make wrong decisions without having all the data. Their solution is to keep the data away, to protect us. Our solution is to get the data, to empower ourselves.

When the people of this country donated their nickels and dimes, their sweat and time, to build community hospitals, they had little idea that 31 million Americans would not have the financial key to get in. Yes, the world of medicine has changed.

Since 1983 the People's Medical Society has been at the forefront of the medical consumerism movement. PMS's sole purpose is to get information to you so that you have the best experience you possibly can in your medical encounters. The People's Medical Society contends that you are your own best advocate and that you can get the most appropriate and best medical care possible with the right tools and information.

This book is designed to be one part of your medical empowerment arsenal. Use it!

Charles B. Inlander
President
People's Medical Society

1

The Key to Translating Medical Terms

As the medical world becomes more specialized and technical (and as new medical "cures" are invented yearly), medical terms appear to multiply overnight. This chapter gives you the key to translating those terms that are not discussed elsewhere in this book—since, by its very nature, this handy publication can only skim the surface, resting momentarily on the most commonly used and crucial-to-know medical terms.

As a rule, medical terms are built from three blocks—the prefixes, roots, and suffixes. Each block doesn't mean much on its own. But when interlocked, these blocks form an infinite number of long and mysterious medical words much favored by white-coated professionals. Fortunately, you don't need the degree of *medicinae doctor* to decode these terms. Just refer to the following translation table to locate the meaning of the blocks and convert them into understandable words and phrases.

First, the prefixes, the blocks that sit at the front of words to indicate the wheres, ifs, and how muches:

a, an = not, without
ab = away from

acid = sour

ad = near (*d* changes to *c, f, g, p, s,* or *t* when it precedes roots that begin with those letters)

alb = white

amphi(i) = both, twice as much

ante = before

anti = against

ap(o) = detached

brady = slow

contra = against, counter to

cry = cold

dia = through or passing through, going apart, between, across

dys = painful, difficult

e = out from

ecto = outside of, outer, exterior

endo = within

epi = upon, on, over

erythr = red

eso = inside

exo = outside of

hemi = half

hyper = increased, excessive, above

hypo = under, below, deficient

in = not (*n* changes to *l, m,* or *r* when it precedes roots that begin with those letters)

infra = below

inter = between

intra = within

leuco, leuko = white

macro = large

mal = bad, ill, wrongful, disordered

meta = after, beyond, changing

micro = small

para = beyond, beside

peri = around
poly = many, multiple
post = after
pre = before, in front of
pseud(o) = false
re = again
retro = backward, behind
sub = under, below
super = above, beyond, over
supra = above
syn (also sy, syl, sym) = with, together
tachy = fast

The next group of blocks, which are called the roots, are at the center of the words. When used in medical terms, the roots usually indicate the body parts affected by a condition:

abdomin = abdomen, stomach
adeno = gland
adip = fat
angi(o) = vessel (blood, lymph)
aph = sense of touch
arteri(o) = artery
arthr(o) = joint
aur = ear
blephar = eyelid
brachi = arm
bronch = windpipe
cardi(o) = heart
cephal = head
cervic = neck
chole, cholo = bile, gall
cholecyst = gallbladder
chondr = cartilage
col(o) = colon

colpo = vagina
crani(o) = skull
cut = skin
cystido, cysto = bladder, sac, cyst
cyto = cell
dent = tooth
enter = intestine
fasci = face
gastr(o) = stomach
glyco = sugar
gnath = jaw
hema, hemato, hemo = blood
hepat(o) = liver
hyster(o) = uterus
ile, ili = intestines, lower abdomen
labi = lip
lact = milk
lapar = loin, flank, abdomen
laryng = windpipe
lipo = fat
lumbar = loin
mast = breast
meno = menstruation
ment = mind
myel = marrow
myelo = spinal cord
myo = muscle
nephro(o) = kidney
neur(o) = nerve
ocul = eye
odont = teeth
oophor = ovary
ophthalm = eye
orchii(o) = testicle
os = mouth, opening

oss, oste(o) = bone
ot(o) = ear
ov = egg
pharyng = throat
phleb = vein
pleur = rib
pneuma, pneumato, pneumo = air, gas, lung
pod = foot
procto = anus, rectum
pulmo = lung
ren = kidney
rhino = nose
salping = fallopian tube
sperm, spermato = semen
splen = spleen
staphyl = uvula
stear = fat
tact = touch
teno = tendon
thorac(o) = chest
thromb = clot, lump
tracheo = windpipe
ur = urine
ureter(o) = tube from kidney to bladder, carrying urine
urethra = tube from bladder to the exterior
vas = vessel, duct
veno = vein
vesic = bladder

Finally, there are the suffixes, the linguistic cabooses that specify what has gone wrong with—or what will be done to—the part of the body designated by a medical word's prefix and root:

algia = pain
blast = a growth in its early stages

cele = tumor, hernia
cente = puncture
desis = fusion
dynia = pain
ectomy = excision of, surgical removal
hydr = water
itis = inflammation
lysis = freeing of
megaly = very large
oma = tumor, swelling
oscopy = looking at an organ or internal part
osis = disease, abnormal condition or process
ostomy = creation of an artificial opening
otomy = incision, cutting into
pathy = disease of, abnormality
pexy = fix, sew
plasty = reconstruct, formation of
pnea = breathing
ptosis = falling, drooping
rhage, rhagia, rrhage, rrhagis = bursting forth, bleeding
rhea, rrhea = flow, discharge
scler(osis) = hard, hardening
uria = urine (condition of, presence in)

Put the blocks together, and they form a medical term. For example, suppose your doctor says that you are suffering from endocarditis. Just consult the lists: prefix "endo" means within; "cardio" has to do with the heart; and "itis" means inflammation. Endocarditis: inflammation of the inside of the heart (more or less). Certainly not a cheery diagnosis, but at least you have the information you need to ask more intelligent questions about what is going to happen to you next.

2

Medical
Abbreviations

Ah, medical abbreviations—those shorthand codes shared by doctors, pharmacists, and nurses as part of a long tradition of cryptic communication that excludes consumers. Medical abbreviations are rampant in medical records and hospital charts, and they are particularly prominent when scrawled across prescription forms. Fortunately for consumers, translating those compacted terms into everyday language is not difficult. All you need is the key. To that end, we give you this table of common medical abbreviations. Note that abbreviations most likely to show up on prescription forms have been highlighted in bold.

a = before
A2 = both ears
aa. = of each
ac = before meals
Ad. = to, up to
AD = right ear
ADL = activities of daily living
ad lib = as needed, as desired
AF = auricular fibrillation

agit = shake, stir
AL = left ear
AM = morning
AMA = against medical advice
Ap. = appendicitis
Aq. = water
ASHD = arteriosclerotic heart disease
BE = barium enema
bid = twice a day
Bl. time = bleeding time
BM = bowel movement
BMR = basal metabolic rate
BP = blood pressure
BRP = bathroom privileges
Bx = biopsy
C = centigrade
$\bar{c}$ = with
CA = cancer
CAD = coronary artery disease
cap(s) = capsule(s)
CBC = complete blood count
CBD = common bile duct
CC = chief complaint
cc = cubic centimeter
CCU = coronary care unit
CHD = coronary heart disease; congenital heart disease
CHF = congestive heart failure
Chol = cholesterol
Cl. time = clotting time
CNS = central nervous system
comp = compound
cont rem = continue the medicine
COPD = chronic obstructive pulmonary disease
CSF = cerebrospinal fluid
CV = cardiovascular

CVA = cerebrovascular accident
CVP = central venous pressure
CXR = chest X ray
d = give
D&C = dilation and curettage
dd in d = from day to day
dec = pour off
dexter = the right
dil = dilute
Disp. = dispense
div = divide
DM = diabetes mellitus
dos = dose
dur dolor = while pain lasts
D/W = dextrose in water
Dx = diagnosis
ECG or EKG = electrocardiogram
EEG = electroencephalogram
emp = as directed
ER = emergency room
ext = for external use
F = Fahrenheit
FBS = fasting blood sugar
febris = fever
FH = family history
Fx = fracture
GA = general anesthesia
garg = gargle
GB = gallbladder
GC = gonorrhea
GI = gastrointestinal
GL = glaucoma
gm = grams
gr = grain(s)
grad = by degrees

gravida = pregnancies
gtt = drops
GTT = glucose tolerance test
GU = genitourinary
GYN = gynecology
h = hour, hourly
HASHD = hypertensive arteriosclerotic heart disease
Hb or Hgb = hemoglobin
HCT = hematocrit
HHD = hypertensive heart disease
HOB = head of bed
HPI = history of present illness
h.s. = at bedtime
Hx = history
$\dot{\text{i}}$ = one
$\ddot{\text{ii}}$ = two
$\dddot{\text{iii}}$ = three
ICU = intensive care unit
I&D = incision and drainage
IM = intramuscular
I.M. = infectious mononucleosis
ind = daily
I&O = intake and output (measure fluids going into and out of body)
IPPB = intermittent positive pressure breathing
IV = intravenous
IVP = intravenous pyelogram
L = left
liq = liquid
LLE = left lower extremity
LLQ = left lower quadrant
LMP = last menstrual period
LP = lumbar puncture
LUE = left upper extremity
LUQ = left upper quadrant

ⓜ = murmur

M = mix

m et n = morning and night

mg = milligram

MI = myocardial infarction (heart attack)

ml = milliliter

mor dict = in the manner directed

MS = mitral stenosis; morphine sulfate; multiple sclerosis

neg. = negative

N-G = nasogastric

no. = number

non rep; nr = do not repeat

NPO = non per os (nothing by mouth)

NS = normal saline

N&V = nausea and vomiting

O_2 = oxygen

o = none

$\bar{o}$ = with

ϕ = without

OD = right eye

O.D. = once a day

OL = left eye

OOB = out of bed

OPD = outpatient department

OR = operating room

OS = left eye

OT = occupational therapy

OU = both eyes

P; $\bar{p}$ = after

Para = number of births

Path. = pathology

pc = after meals

PE = physical examination; pulmonary embolus

PI = present illness

pil = pill

po = orally (by mouth)

Post. = posterior

post-op = postoperative, after the operation

PM = evening

PR = pulse rate

pr = by rectum

prn = as needed, as often as necessary

Prog. = prognosis

pt = patient

PT = physical therapy

PTA = prior to admission

Px = prognosis

q = every

qam = every morning

qd = daily

qh = every hour

q2h = every two hours

q3h = every three hours

q4h = every four hours

q8h = every eight hours

qhs = at hour of sleep

qid = four times a day

qn = every night

qod = every other day

qs = proper amount, quantity sufficient

qv = as much as desired

R = right

rbc = red blood cell

RBC = red blood cell count

rep = repeat

RHD = rheumatic heart disease

RLQ = right lower quadrant

RN = registered nurse

ROM = range of motion

RR = respiratory rate; recovery room

RT = radiation therapy
rub = red
RUQ = right upper quadrant
Rx = prescription; therapy
s̄ = without
S&A = sugar and acetone (a urine test for diabetics)
sc = subcutaneous
Scop. = scopolamine
SH = social history
SICU = surgical intensive care unit
sig = write, let it be imprinted
sing = of each
sl = under the tongue
SOB = shortness of breath
sol = solution
solv = dissolve
SOP = standard operating procedure
SOS = can repeat in emergency
ss = half
SSE = soapsuds enema
stat = right away, immediately
sub Q = subcutaneous
suppos = suppository
susp = suspension
Sx = symptoms
T&A = tonsillectomy and adenoidectomy
tab(s) = tablet(s)
TAT = tetanus antitoxin
tere = rub
TIA = transient ischemic attack
tid = three times a day
tinc. or tinct. = tincture
TPR = temperature, pulse, and respiration
top = apply topically
Tx = treatment

ung = ointment
ungt = ointment
URI = upper respiratory infection
ut dict = as directed
UTI = urinary tract infection
VD = venereal disease
VS = vital signs
WBC = white blood cell count
WC = wheelchair
YO = year old
x = times
↑ = increase
↗ = increasing
↓ = decrease
↙ = decreasing
→ = leads to
← = resulting from
♂ = male
♀ = female

3

And Still More Medical Lingo

The medical profession repeatedly uses certain words that consumers use in everyday life—but the medical world uses those words in a slightly different context. The end result? Confusion and chaos if the consumer is not aware of these hidden meanings. Here are common but crucial medical terms that you are apt to hear when visiting the doctor. These are important to learn, no matter what the state of your health.

Acute. Refers to a condition with symptoms that are severe, develop quickly, and do not last a long time, as opposed to chronic conditions.

Benign. Refers to an abnormal growth that will not spread or recur and that does not endanger life, as opposed to a malignant growth.

Chronic. Refers to a condition with symptoms that last a long time—weeks, months, or years—as opposed to acute conditions.

Congenital. Refers to a condition that is present from birth.

Contagious. Refers to a disease that can spread from one person to another.

Contraindication. A situation or condition under which a drug or medication should never be taken.

Elective surgery. An operation the patient chooses to have on his or her own. It is not an emergency or a medical imperative.

Iatrogenic. Doctor-caused; refers to an illness or condition produced in a patient by the actions of a physician or of medical care.

Idiopathic. Refers to an illness or condition with an unknown cause.

Infarct. An area of tissue that is dead or dying, having been deprived of oxygen by a clot that blocked blood flow. The most common infarctions are cerebral, myocardial or cardiac, and pulmonary.

Invasive. Refers to a procedure that involves cutting through the skin or inserting an object into the body for diagnostic or therapeutic purposes.

Malignant. Refers to a harmful growth (usually cancer) that can spread into surrounding tissue and eventually cause death, as opposed to a benign growth.

Neoplasm. A tumor or a new growth of abnormal tissue (such as cancer) that has much uncontrolled cell multiplication.

Nosocomial. Refers to an infection acquired during hospitalization, produced by microorganisms in the hospital itself.

Palliative. Refers to treatment designed to soothe or provide relief but not to cure.

Pathogen. A disease-producing organism.

Placebo. A substance that has no value in a real therapeutic pharmacological sense, but that helps a patient who believes that it will work. Placebos are often given to patients who psychologically require a pill (and sometimes do well after taking it) or as part of clinical trials to test the effectiveness of new drugs.

Prolapse. The falling down or slippage of a body part from its normal position.

Prosthesis. An artificial part used to replace a missing body part. Artificial limbs and dentures are both examples of prosthetic devices.

Remission. The disappearance of a condition's symptoms for a long or short period of time.

Resection. Surgical removal of a section of an organ or body tissue.

Trauma. A wound or injury to the body or mind.

Urgent. Refers to a condition that must be addressed immediately.

Vital signs. The basic signs of life: temperature, pulse, and respiration rate.

Workup. What is done in a doctor's office or a hospital to get enough information to arrive at a diagnosis. A workup includes taking a medical history, a physical examination, and a variety of lab tests such as blood tests and urinalysis, as well as such things as X rays.

4

Mainstream
M.D. Practitioners

What's in a name? In the world of medical terminology, a physician's title is a clue to the services he or she provides. And what a confusing range of services is available, all delivered by an ever-expanding circle of specialists and subspecialists. An internist, for example, may subspecialize in cardiovascular medicine, critical care medicine, endocrinology, gastroenterology, geriatric medicine, hematology, oncology, nephrology, rheumatology, just to name a few options. If you don't know what all those specialty names mean, don't despair. Here's a helpful guide to who's who among mainstream M.D. practitioners.

Allergist. Diagnoses and treats allergies, asthma cases, and skin problems such as hives and contact dermatitis.

Allopathic physician. Treats diseases with medications and active intervention and according to scientific research. Practitioners who have earned the M.D. degree are considered allopathic physicians.

Anesthesiologist. Dispenses anesthetics and monitors the condition and vital signs of patients undergoing surgery.

Cardiologist. Diagnoses and treats heart disease; may perform cardiac catheterization and pacemaker implantation and administer stress tests and other procedures.

Dentist. Cares for and treats teeth and the surrounding tissue and bone structure of the oral cavity.

Dermatologist. Diagnoses and treats skin problems.

Emergency physician. Deals with the kinds of problems seen in emergency room situations.

Endocrinologist. Diagnoses and treats disorders of the endocrine glands.

Family practitioner. Deals with and oversees the total health care of the individual and his or her family.

Gastroenterologist. Diagnoses and treats problems of the stomach and intestines—the gastrointestinal tract.

Geriatrician. Deals with diseases of the elderly and the problems associated with aging.

Gynecologist. Diagnoses and treats problems associated with the female reproductive organs.

Hematologist. Diagnoses and treats diseases and disorders of the blood and blood-forming parts of the body.

Immunologist. Studies and treats problems of the body's immune system, including allergies, infections, and life-threatening diseases such as AIDS.

Internist. Diagnoses and nonsurgically treats diseases, especially those of adults. Internists may act as highly trained family doctors, or they may subspecialize.

Nephrologist. Deals with diseases of the kidney.

Neurologist. Diagnoses and treats nervous system disorders.

Neurosurgeon. Performs surgery on the nervous system (the brain, spinal cord, and nerves).

Obstetrician. Deals with the medical aspects of and intervention in pregnancy and labor.

Oncologist. Deals with tumors and other cancers; this person may also be a hematologist.

Ophthalmologist. Diagnoses and treats diseases of and injuries to the eye; may perform cataract removals, retina reattachments, and other operations. (This is not the same as an **optometrist.** An optometrist examines the eyes and diagnoses and treats visual problems through the use of lenses, visual aids, and visual therapies, but is not an M.D.)

Orthopedist. Treats and corrects deformities or damage to the musculoskeletal system—bone, muscle, and ligament.

Otolaryngologist. Explores problems and treats disease in the interrelated areas of the ear, nose, and throat; often known as the ENT specialist.

Pathologist. Diagnoses and monitors disease by means of information gathered by lab tests and microscopic examination of tissue, cells, and bodily fluids.

Pediatrician. Diagnoses and treats diseases of childhood and monitors the growth, development, and well-being of preadolescents.

Plastic surgeon. Restores and rebuilds body parts.

Podiatrist. Diagnoses and treats diseases, injuries, deformities, and other conditions of the foot.

Proctologist. Deals with diseases of the anus, rectum, and colon.

Psychiatrist. Examines, treats, and prevents mental illness through noninvasive (psychoanalysis) or pharmaceutical means. (Do not confuse this specialist with the nonphysician psychologist.)

Pulmonologist. Diagnoses and treats diseases of the lungs and chest tissue.

Radiologist. Studies and uses various types of radiation, including X rays, in the diagnosis and treatment of disease.

Reproductive endocrinologist. Deals with problems related to reproduction and infertility.

Rheumatologist. Diagnoses and treats inflammation, deterioration, and other problems (such as arthritis) having to do with the joints and connective tissues.

Thoracic surgeon. Performs operations on the heart and major vessels and the lungs; may also perform surgical procedures on the trachea and esophagus and on hiatal hernias.

Urologist. Diagnoses and treats diseases of the urinary system as well as the male reproductive organs.

NOTE: We mentioned earlier that a physician's title is a clue to the services he or she provides. We stress the word *clue.* Why? In most of the United States, M.D.'s can call themselves whatever they want. That means medical practitioners can claim to have expertise in an area in which they have no medical certification or training—in effect "self-designating" their area of specialization. You would be wise to discuss a doctor's qualifications before using his or her services. While certification and specialization *do not guarantee* that the doctor has the right combination of knowledge, experience, and skills to give you the kind of care you need, certification and specialization can serve as a yardstick for evaluating and selecting a practitioner.

Nontraditional Therapies

The search for the best health care may take you to alternative health care services and nontraditional therapies. Since these services are not part of the mainstream medical system, their names may be unfamiliar. Here's an alphabetical walk-through of the array of alternative health therapies.

Acupressure. A system of medicine that addresses health problems through use of the fingertips to apply pressure and thus stimulate acupressure points along "meridians" found on the body. Also known as shiatsu.

Acupuncture. The use of very thin needles inserted under the skin in order to treat illness and restore good health. Acupuncturists often make use of herbal medicine, nutritional measures, relaxation skills, and exercise.

Alexander technique. A therapy that attempts to correct disorders by improving posture.

Ayurvedic medicine. An ancient system of holistic medicine that works on the premise that disease is caused by imbalances in the body's five basic elements—earth, fire, water, air, and ether—and the forces in those elements. Branches of ayurvedic medicine include surgery, obstetrics, gynecology, pediatrics, and psychology.

Biofeedback. The use of the conscious mind to control the involuntary body functions (such as respiration, heartbeat, and body temperature) to address health disorders, chronic pain, and stress.

Chiropractic. The manipulation of the vertebrae as a method of restoring health. A chiropractor holds the degree of Doctor of Chiropractic (D.C.). Chiropractors from the "straight school" only use traditional spinal manipulation. Chiropractors from the "mixed school," who account for the majority of chiropractors in practice today, also use adjunctive therapies such as heat, ultrasound, traction, vitamins, minerals, and exercise.

Christian healing. A therapy based on the belief that a healer has the power to cure physical illnesses through the laying-on of hands.

Feldenkrais technique. A technique that stresses body and health awareness through movement and private manipulative (massage) treatment.

Herbal medicine. The use of herbal mixtures—considered to be free of the harmful side effects of modern medicines—to prevent and cure illnesses.

Homeopathic medicine. The use of natural medicines in treating illness to stimulate a person's own healing process while avoiding harmful side effects. Homeopathic physicians believe that medicines that cause symptoms of diseases in healthy people will bring about cures in sick people, and they believe that medications should never be used in combination. Most homeopathic physicians in practice today are M.D.'s or D.O.'s who have additional training in homeopathic principles.

Hydrotherapy. The use of water for the treatment of certain illnesses and/or bodily injuries. Hydrotherapy includes the whirlpool bath, swimming, ice pack, sitz bath, contrast baths, cold mitten friction, Epsom salt bath, and colonics.

Hypnotherapy. A therapy often used in the treatment of physical and mental disorders, such as helping patients deal with pain from deep burn wounds, migraine headaches, chronic pain, stress, stomach problems, arthritis, colitis, and hemophilia.

Kinesiology. The use of therapeutic touch to correct imbalances in the body's energy system and restore health. Kinesiologists are trained in the proper functioning of the body's muscle systems. Chiropractors and massage therapists sometimes use the principles of kinesiology.

Massage therapy. The use of massage (hand manipulation of the body) to create a feeling of relaxation, ease mental and physical tension, alleviate aches and pains, improve circulation, and generally reinvigorate and stimulate the body's systems. Forms of massage therapy include Swedish massage, shiatsu, acupressure, rolfing, reflexology, polarity, and bioenergetics.

Midwifery. The art of assisting in childbirth. Midwives generally are certified nurse-midwives, registered nurses who have taken additional training in obstetrics-gynecology and newborn care and who have passed a credentialing examination from the American College of Nurse-Midwives.

Myotherapy. A method of pain relief that is based upon locating "trigger points" in muscles that cause the muscles to go into spasm. Using the fingers, knuckles, or elbows, a myotherapist applies pressure to these trigger points. The myotherapists with the most rigorous training are the Bonnie Prudden Certified Myotherapists.

Naturopathic medicine. A system of medicine that emphasizes the natural healing forces that are present in the body and makes use of massage, light, heat, air, and water in therapy. Naturopathic physicians complete courses in traditional naturopathic philosophy, medical science, and natural therapeutics to earn the degree of Doctor of Naturopathic Medicine (N.D.).

Orthomolecular medicine. A system of medicine that emphasizes the use of large doses or megadoses of vitamins to treat illness and emphasizes dietary changes as a way of improving the body's nutrient intake.

Osteopathic medicine. A system of medicine that considers the entire body when treating disease. An osteopathic physician uses manipulative therapy to reposition the joints in the body or the vertebrae of the spine, and makes use of the same methods of diagnosis and treatment as mainstream allopathic (M.D.) practitioners—namely, examinations, tests, X rays, medications, and surgery. Practitioners complete four years of study to be granted the degree of Doctor of Osteopathy (D.O.); some become board certified by the American Osteopathic Association.

Reflexology. The stimulation of certain areas of the feet that correspond to various organs and other parts of the body. Proper stimulation of these points can aid in maintaining good health. Reflexologists may be certified, which indicates they have completed a formal course of instruction in reflexology.

Rolfing. A form of deep muscle massage that creates structural balances in the body. Some massage therapists, kinesiologists, and chiropractors are also familiar with rolfing.

Yoga. An ancient philosophy of life that espouses the uniting of the body, mind, and spirit to achieve higher self-realization and better health. Forms of yoga include hatha, mantra, bhakti, jnana, karma, raja, and laya.

NOTE: Not every type of alternative health care service may be licensed in your state. If the state does license and regulate a particular practice, all this means is that minimum standards have been met, probably education credentials. If particular practices are not licensed, it does not necessarily mean they are not legitimate, but it means you need to be diligent about checking credentials yourself. To find out whether these are licensed, call your state's department of occupational and professional licensing.

Hospital Health Professionals

Anyone who has been in the hospital knows that you see far more of other staff members' faces than that of your doctor. In fact, you can count yourself among the fortunate if you see your doctor once a day. Here's a look at the types of medical people who may parade past your bed in the course of your stay.

Adult nurse practitioner. A registered nurse with advanced, specialized training in the primary care of adults.

Anesthetist. A person who administers anesthetics for surgery and diagnostic procedures. May be a nurse-anesthetist or an anesthesia technician.

Certified nurse-midwife. A registered nurse who has additional advanced training in childbirth and the care of pregnant women and who has passed a nurse-midwifery certification examination.

Family nurse practitioner. A registered nurse with advanced, specialized training in the primary care of adults and family members.

Gerontological nurse. A nurse who cares for older patients.

House staff. Doctors in training in a hospital, plus hospital-based physicians, who are the primary physicians for patients without personal physicians and who assist in the care of those who do.

Intern. A doctor in the first year of postgraduate training in a hospital. The term is being replaced by "first-year resident."

Licensed practical nurse (LPN) or licensed vocational nurse (LVN). A person who has undergone training in a vocational technical setting, hospital program, or community college and has been granted a license to provide general care to the sick. Considered less well trained than a registered nurse, but functions may overlap considerably, depending on state laws. Often reports to registered nurses.

Maternal-gynecological-neonatal nurse. A nurse who cares for mothers and newborn infants.

Medical-surgical nurse. A nurse who cares for adults with chronic illnesses and for presurgical and postsurgical patients.

Medical technician. A person with training that allows him or her to carry out some of the functions of holders of the M.D. or D.O. degree, especially in emergency and life-support situations outside of hospitals and during transport to hospitals. May be more highly trained in their limited areas of expertise than nurse practitioners or physician assistants.

Nurse practitioner (NP). A registered nurse who has taken additional training and is certified to handle some of the functions of a holder of the M.D. or D.O. degree.

Nurses' aide. A person who assists trained nurses in a hospital by performing nonspecialized tasks.

Nutritionist. A person who teaches people about nutrition and helps people plan meals tailored to their particular health and dietary needs.

Occupational therapist. A person who uses creative activity as a therapy for helping patients recover or rehabilitate from illness, injury, or disability. May have completed an accredited program in occupational therapy and passed a professional examination.

Orderly. A person who does the hospital's routine or heavy work, such as cleaning, moving supplies, and moving patients.

Paramedic. A technician trained and skilled in the delivery of medical care in emergency situations.

Patients' representative. A person employed by the hospital to mediate between patients and hospital staff. Ideally, this person acts as a patient rights activist, dispensing information to patients and getting complaints resolved.

Pediatric nurse practitioner. A registered nurse who has advanced, specialized training in the nursing care of children.

Pharmacist. A person who has graduated from an accredited school of pharmacy and passed a state board examination. Assures safety, efficacy, and efficiency in obtaining, storing, prescribing, dispensing, delivering, administering, and using drugs and related articles. Often maintains medication profiles on patients receiving prescriptions to reduce adverse reactions, allergies, and contraindicated use of drugs.

Physical therapist. A person who has been trained and licensed in physical therapy, primarily to help people rehabilitate from injuries or diseases affecting muscles, joints, nerves, and bones. Works under the direction of a physician.

Physician assistant. A person trained to carry out some of the functions of holders of the M.D. or D.O. degree. May have more training than a nurse practitioner or a medical technician. Works under physicians' supervision.

Physician extender. A term that refers to people who have been trained to do part of what a holder of the M.D. or D.O. degree can do. Physician extenders include nurse practitioners, physician assistants, and medical technicians. They are used heavily in health maintenance organizations.

Private duty nurse. A nurse who is hired to care for one patient exclusively in a hospital or nursing home and is paid directly by the patient or his or her family.

Psychiatric and mental health nurse. A person who cares for patients with mental and emotional disorders.

Radiotherapist. A person who treats cancer and other diseases using X rays and radioactive substances.

Registered dietitian (RD). A person with education in nutrition who has passed a national registration exam and who plans and directs food service programs in medical care facilities such as hospitals.

Registered nurse (RN). Generally, a highly trained nurse, one licensed by a state to provide general nursing services after passing a qualifying examination. Three types of nursing education lead to registered-nurse licenses: two-year community college programs, three-year hospital-affiliated diploma programs, and four-year baccalaureate-degree programs.

Resident. A doctor taking postgraduate training in a hospital, often working towards certification in a specialty area.

Social worker. A person, usually with a Master's of Social Work (M.S.W.) degree and sometimes with certification, who works with people who are ill, disabled, aged, or handicapped to help them adjust to disabilities or cope with long-term illness.

Speech pathologist. A person, usually with a postgraduate degree, who works with people who have communicative disorders resulting from total or partial hearing loss, brain injury, cleft palate, voice pathology, learning disabilities, mental retardation, emotional problems, and so on. (Although the two practitioners often work together, a speech pathologist is not to be confused with an **audiologist**, who assesses and treats hearing problems, sometimes by fitting and dispensing hearing aids.)

7

Health Care Facilities

It used to be that when you wanted medical or health care, you hopped on down to the doctor's office, visited the hospital emergency room, or got checked into the local hospital. Today those health care options exist—and many more. New types of health care settings have sprung up, all vying for your medical dollars. This is one instance where you need to know what the name of each type of facility means—so that you know what you're literally getting into.

Ambulatory. Refers to a facility that treats patients on an outpatient basis; a walk-in or drop-in center. It may be a freestanding center or may be part of a hospital.

Childbirth center. A freestanding childbirth facility staffed by nurse-midwives.

Custodial care facility. A nursing home that provides round-the-clock room and board to aged or handicapped persons who require personal care, supervision, or assistance in daily activity.

Emergicenter. A freestanding emergency center.

Freestanding center. An independent medical facility, one not affiliated with a hospital.

General hospital. A hospital that provides diagnostic and treatment services for surgical and nonsurgical conditions.

Hospice. A facility that provides medical care in a homelike setting for the terminally ill.

Intermediate care facility. A nursing home that provides health care and services to persons who do not require the care and services of a hospital or a skilled nursing facility.

Nonprofit voluntary hospital. An entity organized to provide hospital services on a nonprofit and nongovernmental basis, generally with alleged oversight from the community they serve by means of self-perpetuating boards of trustees. The classic American hospital.

Proprietary or private hospital. A hospital owned and operated by corporations or individuals (such as doctors) as a profit-making business.

Recovery care center. A facility that provides up to three days of postsurgical care in a hotellike environment for patients who have had elective surgery. No emergency or acute care services are provided.

Rehabilitation facility. A facility that provides medical, health-related, social, and/or vocational services to disabled persons to help them attain their maximum functional capacity; may operate independently or as a satellite facility associated with a hospital.

Skilled nursing facility. A nursing home that provides skilled nursing care and related services for seriously ill patients who require inpatient medical or nursing care similar to that received in a hospital. Skilled nursing is distinguished from intermediate care and custodial care, which may meet some minor medical needs but are intended primarily to support elderly and disabled individuals in the tasks of daily living. However, not all patients in a skilled nursing facility are necessarily assigned skilled nursing care.

Special care unit. Portion of a hospital organized and staffed to take care of one kind of (usually serious) problem, such as a cardiac care unit, an intensive care unit, or a burn unit.

Specialty hospital. A hospital that only admits people with particular illnesses or conditions.

Surgicenter. A freestanding surgical center.

Veterans Administration (VA) hospital. Hospital care in Veterans Administration facilities is provided to any veteran, providing he or she meets specific criteria: for example, the veteran is rated "service connected"; or is retired from active duty for a disability incurred or aggravated while in military service; or is in receipt of a VA pension; or is in need of care for a condition possibly related to exposure to dioxin or other toxic substance while in Vietnam between 1964 and 1975; and so on.

Tools of the Medical Trade

Every trade has its tools of craftsmanship, and the medical profession is no exception. Doctors use their instruments, tools, and devices hundreds of times during the course of the workweek. Consumers, however, are less frequently exposed to those everyday medical appliances and thus are often unacquainted with—and intimidated by—the numerous metallic and sometimes mechanical devices of foreign name and unknown purpose. Here's an introduction to common tools of the medical trade.

Anesthesia machine. A device that delivers anesthesia gas to the patient during surgery.

Apnea monitor. A machine that detects breathing problems (apnea) in infants and sounds an alarm when an infant's breathing or heart rate slows or stops.

Aspirator. A tube with vacuum suction that is used to remove fluid, tissue, or other substances from the body.

Balloon. An inflatable device inserted in the body, often by means of a catheter, that is used to dilate (widen) a passageway.

Bougie. A thin, flexible instrument, either hollow or solid, that is inserted into a narrow passageway to explore, measure, or dilate (widen) that area. Pronounced *boo-zhe.*

Bronchoscope. An endoscope that is inserted down the throat to the lungs to examine air passages.

Catheter. A flexible tube that is inserted into a vein or artery to withdraw liquid or air or to inject a substance.

Colposcope. An instrument with a magnifying lens that is inserted in the vagina to examine the interior.

Cryoprobe. An instrument that applies extreme cold to tissue to freeze and destroy growths.

Curette. A small surgical rod with a sharp-edged loop at one end, used in performing dilation and curettage (D&C).

Cystoscope. An endoscope used to examine the bladder.

Defibrillator. A device that uses brief electroshocks to counter-act abnormal flutters of the heart (called fibrillation) and restore a normal pattern of heartbeats.

Endoscope. A long, flexible fiberoptic tube that enables a physician to look into a body cavity, photograph the interior, and take a tissue sample. Endoscopes used in different parts of the body have different names.

Endotracheal tube. A tube placed in the windpipe by way of the nose or mouth; used in conjunction with a ventilator or respirator to provide artificial breathing.

Funduscope. See **ophthalmoscope.**

Heart-lung machine. A machine into which the bloodstream is diverted for oxygenation and pumping during heart surgery.

Hemodialyzer. A machine that pumps blood through a membrane (filter) to remove the impurities in the blood that have built up because of a malfunctioning kidney.

Intravenous (IV) administration set. An elevated container with a long tube that is inserted into a vein; used to slowly infuse intravenous liquids (which may include vitamins, minerals, salt, sugar, protein, and antibiotics) into the bloodstream. Sometimes referred to as a drip.

Laser. A surgical tool using an intense, high-energy beam of light that can be tightly focused to vaporize, cut, or fuse body tissues.

Medical linear accelerator. A computerized machine that delivers radiation doses.

Nasogastric tube. A tube passed into the stomach by way of the mouth; used to empty the stomach or to feed the patient.

Nebulizer. A device that acts as an atomizer, mixing a drug with water to produce a mist that can be inhaled.

Ophthalmoscope. An instrument with mirrors and lenses that is used to view the tissues of the interior of the eye.

Otoscope. An instrument for examining the interior of the ear.

Oxygen tent or cone. A canopy erected around a person that delivers a steady flow of oxygen to prevent tissue damage due to oxygen deficiency.

Peak-flow meter. An instrument that measures how much air a person can forcibly exhale from the lungs; used to determine lung efficiency.

Proctoscope. An instrument with a source of lighting that is used to examine the rectum.

Respirator. See **ventilator.**

Retractor. A surgical instrument that separates organs and tissues and holds them apart.

Scalpel. A small surgical knife with a straight handle and thin blade.

Sigmoidoscope. An endoscope used to inspect the colon.

Speculum. An instrument that opens a body cavity wider so that the inside of the opening can be seen more clearly.

Sphygmomanometer. An instrument that measures blood pressure and gives a systolic reading (the measurement of blood pressure when the left ventricle contracts and the blood's force against the vessel is at its greatest strength) and a diastolic reading (the measurement of blood pressure when the heart is at rest). The sphygmomanometer is commonly called a blood pressure cuff and is used in conjunction with a stethoscope.

Spirometer. A machine that measures and records the volume of air inhaled, the volume exhaled, and the rate of exhalation.

Stethoscope. An instrument for listening to the activity of parts of the body, particularly the lungs and heart. A metal disc placed on the body picks up the body's interior sounds, which the practitioner listens to through the stethoscope's earpieces.

Suture. The thread that is used in sewing up wounds or incisions. Stitches made from suture thread are also known as sutures.

Thermograph. A device that detects and records the amount of heat generated by a body area.

Thorascope. An endoscope that is used for examining the cavity that holds the lungs.

Tonometer. An instrument that measures the pressure inside the eye.

Vaporizer. A device that produces an aerosol or mist.

Ventilator. An artificial breathing machine that regularly pumps air in and out of the lungs. Also called a respirator.

CHAPTER

9

Diagnostic Tests

The medical world loves tests and procedures. You know the scenario: You go to the doctor with a particular complaint, make your case, and then the doctor brusquely tells you what she is going to "do"—only the litany of tests and procedures that she recites sounds more like a curse than a cure. Naturally, before you can give your yea or nay to these tests and procedures, you need to know what they mean. To that end, we've defined the diagnostic tests and procedures most loved by medical practitioners today.

Amniocentesis. A sampling of the amniotic fluid that surrounds the fetus; used to detect certain birth defects and brain and blood disorders.

Angiogram. An X-ray picture of a blood vessel made after injecting an opaque substance or dye through a thin tube (catheter) into blood vessels to make them visible on X-ray film. An angiogram of the arteries is called **arteriogram;** of the veins, **venogram** or **phlebogram;** of the lymph vessels, **lymph-angiogram;** of the heart's arteries, **coronary angiogram.**

Arteriogram. An X-ray picture; used to locate blockages in the arteries. See **angiogram.**

Arthrogram. An X-ray picture of a joint; used to detect injury or damage.

Arthroscopy. An examination of a joint by means of a long, flexible viewing tube inserted into the joint; used to detect injury or damage.

Barium enema. X-ray pictures of the large intestine (colon) made after injecting barium sulfate into the rectum; used to locate abnormalities in the colon. Often called a lower GI (gastrointestinal) series.

Barium meal. X-ray pictures of the esophagus, stomach, and duodenum (first part of the small intestine) made after the patient swallows barium sulfate on an empty stomach. Used to locate problems or abnormalities. Often called an upper GI (gastrointestinal) series.

Biopsy. The removal of a small portion of body tissue for microscopic analysis; often used to check growths that might be cancerous.

Bronchoscopy. An examination of the bronchi (air passages) of the lungs with a flexible, fiberoptic viewing tube that has been inserted down the throat.

Cardiac catheterization. The insertion of a thin, flexible tube (a catheter) through a vein or artery into the heart. Used to collect information about the heart's structure and performance and to inject an opaque substance or dye so that an X ray can be made.

Carotid or cerebral arteriogram. An X-ray picture of the blood vessels of the brain; used in diagnosing stroke. See **angiogram.**

Cholesterol test. A sampling of the blood to determine the amount of cholesterol in the blood.

Colonoscopy. An examination of the colon with a flexible, fiberoptic viewing tube.

Complete blood cell count (CBC). An examination of blood samples to get a count of the number of red cells, white cells, and hemoglobin in the blood and to determine the percentage of red cells in the blood. Used to check for infection or screen for blood disorders.

Computerized axial tomography (CAT) scan. A highly detailed picture of internal body parts constructed by a computer from hundreds of X rays; frequently used to locate disease, tumors, or abnormalities in the selected part of the body.

Coronary angiogram. An X-ray picture of the heart's arteries. Coronary angiography is a form of cardiac catheterization.

Cystogram. An X ray of the bladder made by inserting a thin tube through the urethra into the bladder.

Dilation and curettage (D&C). The removal of a layer of tissue from the wall of the uterus; as a diagnostic test, it is used to diagnose the cause of excessive bleeding or other problems.

Echocardiogram. An ultrasound recording of the heart's internal structures; used to locate heart valve problems or heart deformities.

Electrocardiogram (ECG or EKG). A recording of the heart muscle's activity that is collected by electrodes placed on the body. Used to detect heart damage, as after a heart attack, and to monitor the effect of certain drugs.

Electroencephalogram (EEG). A recording of the brain's electrical impulses and brain patterns that is collected by electrodes placed on the scalp. Often used to detect brain damage, diagnose epilepsy, or confirm brain death.

Electromyogram (EMG). A recording of the electrical activity of resting and contracting muscles that is collected by an electrode and a thin needle attached to the skin. Used to detect weakness, paralysis, or other problems in the muscle.

Hysterosalpingogram. An X-ray picture of the uterus and fallopian tubes.

Lower gastrointestinal (GI) series. See **barium enema.**

Magnetic resonance imaging (MRI). The use of a magnetic field (instead of radiation) to produce detailed, computer-generated pictures of the body.

Mammogram. An X-ray picture of the breast; used to diagnose certain conditions, including breast cancer.

Myelogram. An X-ray picture of the fluid-filled space around the spinal cord; used to locate tumors, nerve injuries, and slipped discs.

Pap test. A sampling of the tissue of the cervix; used to detect abnormal cells and cancer. Also called a cervical smear.

Positron emission tomography (PET). A technique for making computer-generated images of the brain or other body organs by means of radioactive isotopes injected into the body; used to locate abnormal tissue.

Sigmoidoscopy. A nonsurgical examination of the colon by means of a long, flexible viewing tube.

Spinal tap. A sampling of cerebrospinal fluid removed from the spinal canal by means of a long needle; used to diagnose diseases of and injuries to the brain and spinal cord, especially in suspected cases of meningitis and stroke.

Thermogram. A photograph of the surfaces of the body made by a camera with heat-sensitive film; often used to detect varicose veins and breast tumors.

Ultrasound scan. A picture of organs and structures deep inside the body that has been made with high-frequency sound waves. Used to gather information about some part of the body; also used on pregnant women to gain information about the health or development of the fetus.

Upper gastrointestinal (GI) series. See **barium meal.**

Venogram. An X-ray picture of the interior of a vein. See **angiogram.**

X ray. A picture of the body's internal structures made with electromagnetic rays with a short wavelength.

The Most Frequent Inpatient Procedures

Just as the names given to medical tests are puzzling to people outside the medical trade, so too are the names of the surgical procedures that often follow on the heels of those tests. This chapter describes the top 25 most frequently performed inpatient surgeries, as enumerated by the medical newspaper *HealthWeek* (February 25, 1991). More than 5.6 million of these surgical procedures were performed in hospitals in 1989, according to that publication. *HealthWeek*'s list of common surgeries forms the framework for this section. To each entry we've added a definition—in the language of consumers, of course.

1. **Cervical cesarean section.** Delivery of a child through an incision in the lower part of the mother's abdomen and uterus.
2. **Total cholecystectomy.** Gallbladder removal.
3. **Abdominal hysterectomy.** Surgical removal of the uterus, fallopian tubes, ovaries, and sometimes the lymphatic glands by means of an incision through the lower abdomen.
4. **Left cardiac catheterization.** The passing of a thin, flexible tube (called a catheter) through a vein or artery

into one of the heart's chambers; used to collect blood samples and information about the heart's structure and performance.

5. **Repair of obstetric laceration.** Surgical repair of tears in tissue that occurred during childbirth.

6. **Transurethral prostatectomy.** Removal of part of the prostate gland; also known as transurethral resection of the prostate (TURP).

7. **Intervertebral disc excision.** Removal of a disc from the spine.

8. **Appendectomy.** Removal of the appendix.

9. **Forceps delivery with episiotomy.** Delivery of a child with the use of sterile forceps applied to the head of the child and with a small incision made in the vagina.

10. **Balloon angioplasty.** The widening of coronary arteries that have been made narrow by a buildup of fat (called plaque). A thin tube (a catheter) with an inflatable balloon is passed into the clogged artery, and the balloon is inflated to compress the plaque against the artery wall, thus making it wider.

11. **Biopsy of esophagus, stomach, and/or duodenum.** The removal for the purpose of analysis of a small sample of tissue from the esophagus (the muscular tube that carries food from the throat to the stomach), the stomach, and/or the duodenum (the first part of the small intestine).

12. **Open reduction of fracture with internal fixation (femur).** Realignment (known as reduction) of a fractured or broken thighbone (femur) by attaching metal screws, nails or plates to hold the broken ends in place.

13. **Combined right/left heart catheterization.** The passing of a thin, flexible tube (called a catheter) through a vein or artery into both of the heart's chambers; used to collect blood samples or check for information about the heart's structure and performance.

14. **Cystoscopy.** Examination of bladder with cystoscope.

15. **Vacuum extraction with episiotomy.** Delivery of a child by means of a suction device and a small cut at the bottom of the vagina.

16. **Wound debridement.** Removal of dead tissue and dirt and debris from a wound.

17. **Vaginal hysterectomy.** Surgical removal of the cervix or the uterus by means of an incision made around and above the cervix.

18. **Open reduction of fracture with internal fixation (tibia/fibula).** Realignment (known as reduction) of a fractured or broken bone in the lower leg by attaching metal screws, nails or plates to hold the broken ends in place.

19. **Venous catheterization.** Insertion of a thin, flexible tube (called a catheter) into a major vein to gather information about the circulatory system or to dispense nutrients or medicines.

20. **Knee replacement.** Surgical replacement of the knee with a man-made replacement.

21. **Unilateral simple mastectomy.** Removal of one breast without removal of the pectoral muscles beneath it or removal of the nearby lymph nodes.

22. **Contrast myelogram.** An X-ray picture of the spine by means of the insertion of a contrast material into the spinal canal.

23. **Dilation & curettage (D&C), postdelivery.** Cleansing of the uterus and removal of birth matter from the uterus following delivery of a child.

24. **Fetal monitoring, intrauterine.** The attachment of a tiny electrode to an unborn baby's scalp (through the mother's vagina) to measure his or her well-being during labor and to detect early signs of potential problems.

25. **Closed biopsy of large bowel.** The removal for analysis of a small sample of tissue from the large bowel via a long, flexible fiberoptic tube.

The Most Frequent Outpatient Procedures

Not all diagnostic tests or surgical procedures are done inside the hospital. An increasing number of procedures are done on an outpatient, or "ambulatory," basis, which means that the patient comes in the day of the procedure, checks out on the same day, and recuperates at home. These are the top eight ambulatory procedures as specified by *Hospital Market Notes*. To each entry we've added a definition—in the language of consumers, of course.

Diagnostic dilation & curettage (D&C). Removal of a layer of tissue from the wall of the uterus to find the cause of a problem, such as excessive bleeding.

Cystoscopy. Examination of the bladder with a type of endoscope known as a cystoscope.

Myringectomy. Insertion of a fine needle into the eardrum to drain fluid and to insert a tiny plastic tube that will let air enter and dry out the middle ear; used to treat severe or recurrent ear infections.

Biopsy of breast tissue. Removal of a small piece of breast tissue, usually gathered to determine whether an abnormal growth in the breast is cancerous.

Local excision of lesion. Removal from the skin of an abnormal tissue or growth such as a cyst, wart, or mole.

Diagnostic laparoscopy. Examination of the inside of the abdomen with a type of endoscope called a laparoscope.

Cataract removal. Surgical removal of a cataract (an opacity in the internal lens of the eye) from the eye, often followed by implantation of an artificial lens.

Relief of carpal tunnel syndrome. Surgery to remove pressure on the nerve in the wrist.

12

Dental Terms

Professionals in the dental field use all of the terms that make up medical language—plus they have a few specialized terms of their own.

Abscess. An area of infection in the mouth that has become a pus-filled inflammation.

Apicoectomy. A treatment for chronic tooth abscesses by cutting out an infected root tip and filling the remaining part of the root.

Appliance. A device, such as braces or retainers, used to slowly move the teeth into alignment.

Bicuspids. Teeth between the canines and the molars that are used to grind and crush food. Also known as **premolars.**

Bite. The way the upper and lower teeth come together when the mouth is closed. Also known as **occlusion.**

Bite-wing X rays. A series of X rays of the teeth made with small pieces of X-ray film that are gripped between the teeth.

Braces. A device that is attached to the teeth and that uses pressure to move teeth into a better alignment.

Bridge. One or several artificial teeth that are cemented in place between natural teeth; used to fill the gap caused by one or more missing teeth.

Calculus. A hard white or brown deposit that forms on the teeth and is built of layers of hardened plaque.

Canines. Teeth at the front of the mouth that are used to cut food.

Caries. Tooth decay; cavities.

Crown. A tooth-shaped shell made of porcelain, gold, or an alloy that is used to cover a broken, decayed, or severely discolored tooth.

Dentifrice. A material, such as toothpaste, that is used to scrub plaque and food particles off the teeth.

Dentin. The part of the tooth that surrounds the pulp, or center of the tooth, and that is encased in enamel.

Dentures. A set of artificial or false teeth that replaces missing teeth.

Enamel. The hard, shiny white substance on the outside of the tooth.

Endodontics. The treatment of diseased or dead teeth.

Extraction. Removal of a tooth.

Filling. Material made of silver or a metal alloy that is used to fill the spot where a cavity had existed before being removed.

Gingivectomy. Removal of diseased areas of the gums around the teeth.

Gingivitis. Inflamed and swollen gums.

Incisors. Teeth at the front of the mouth that are used to cut food.

Malocclusion. Irregularly spaced teeth that result in a faulty occlusion, or bad bite.

Molars. Squarish teeth at the back of the mouth that grind and crush food.

Occlusion. The way the upper and lower teeth fit together when the mouth is closed.

Orthodontics. Dentistry that deals with the jaws and teeth and corrects irregularities of the teeth, sometimes through oral surgery or through the use of such devices as braces and dentures.

Periodontal disease. Disease of the gum caused by gingivitis. Also known as **periodontitis.**

Periodontal pack. A protective coating placed on the gum line after gum surgery to help the gums heal.

Plaque. A potentially damaging coating on the teeth made up of food particles, mucus, and bacteria.

Premolars. Teeth between the canines and the molars that are used to grind and crush food. Also known as **bicuspids.**

Prophylaxis. The cleaning and polishing of teeth.

Pyorrhea. Inflammation of the gums. See **periodontal disease.**

Retainer. A device that fits in the mouth to hold teeth in their new position; usually used after braces have moved the teeth.

Root canal. A procedure for treating a dead tooth—one in which healthy pulp has been replaced with bacteria and decayed pulp. The bacteria in the root canal is cleaned out and destroyed, and the root canal is filled.

Wisdom teeth. The last molars to erupt in the mouth. Not all people have wisdom teeth.

13

Health Insurance Terms

It's bad enough that the medical profession has its own brand of gibberish. But not long after you've left the doctor's office, or passed through a hospital's doors, you're expected to be conversant in another kind of lingo—health insurance-speak. Instead of saying things the simple, comprehensive way, insurance companies feel compelled to dream up a system of cumbersome codes that only their initiates understand. Well, the word is out: Consumers have deciphered those codes. Here, in straightforward language, are the meanings of common health insurance terms.

Accumulation period. The number of days during which the insured person must incur eligible medical expenses at least equal to the deductible in order to receive a benefit.

Allocated benefits. Benefits for which the maximum amount payable for specific services is itemized in the insurance contract.

Ambulatory surgical center. A medical facility that performs outpatient surgical procedures.

Application. A signed statement of facts that an insurance company uses to decide whether to sell you a policy.

Assignment. The insurance company's direct payment (assigning) of benefits to a practitioner or a medical facility instead of making payment through you.

Benefits. What the insurance company agrees to pay when you file a claim.

Cancellation. The termination of a policy before it would normally expire.

Claim. A notification by you, your doctor, or your hospital to your insurance company stating that you have received a medical service and are requesting payment in accordance with the policy.

Coinsurance/copayment. The portion or percentage of the costs of medical services that you, the policyholder, must pay.

Conditionally renewable clause. A provision that permits a policyholder to renew a policy up to a certain age limit, such as 65, provided all conditions of the insurance contract have been met.

Conversion clause. A provision in a group policy that provides the insured person with the opportunity to purchase individual coverage in the event the group policy is terminated.

Coordination of benefits. A practice insurance companies use to avoid duplication of payment when a person is covered by more than one policy.

Covered expense. A medical expense that you incur and the insurance company agrees to pay.

Custodial care facility. A facility that provides round-the-clock room and board to aged or handicapped persons who require personal care, supervision, or assistance in daily activity.

Deductible. The amount you, the policyholder, must pay before an insurance plan pays for any portion of the cost.

Disability insurance. Insurance that pays you a portion of your salary when you are sick or injured and unable to work.

Disease-specific insurance. Insurance that provides benefits should you develop a specific illness such as cancer, heart disease, poliomyelitis, encephalitis, or spinal meningitis.

Effective date. The date insurance begins; the first day you can file a claim and have benefits paid.

Exclusions. Conditions or circumstances that the insurance policy will not cover.

Explanation of benefits. A statement from an insurance company itemizing the medical services you received and the amount of insurance coverage provided for each service.

First-dollar coverage. A policy with no deductible that covers the first dollar of your expenses.

Grace period. A period of time (usually 30 or 31 days) after the date a premium is due during which the policy remains in force and the premium may still be paid without penalty.

Group insurance. Insurance, usually issued through employers and unions, that covers a group of persons.

Guaranteed renewable clause. A provision that guarantees the policyholder the right to renew as long as premiums are paid on time. While the insurance is in force, the company cannot raise the premium unless all policyholders have their premiums raised at the same time.

Health maintenance organization (HMO). An organization that provides a wide range of medical services for a specified group at a fixed monthly payment.

Home health care. Care rendered in a patient's home, such as nursing services, therapy, or medications.

Hospital insurance. Insurance that covers costs of hospital care resulting from injury or illness.

Indemnity policy. Insurance that pays a specified amount of money each day or week that you are in the hospital and that pays a set amount for medical and surgical procedures.

Individual insurance. A policy that you purchase yourself and that is not part of a group plan. The policy covers you and, usually, your dependents.

Individual practice association (IPA). A prepaid health care plan that is offered to groups of people by physicians in private practice.

Inpatient. Someone who is admitted to the hospital for medical services.

Inside limit. A provision that limits insurance payment for any type of service, regardless of the actual cost of the service.

Intermediate care facility. A facility that provides health care and services to persons who do not require the care and services of a hospital or a skilled nursing facility.

Lapsed policy. An insurance policy that has been canceled for nonpayment of premiums.

Major medical insurance. Insurance that offsets the large expenses of a severe and prolonged illness or injury.

Medicaid. A government program that provides assistance to the poor.

Medical-surgical insurance. Insurance that covers some of the fees of physicians and surgeons for care provided in the hospital, office, or home and covers part of the cost of laboratory tests performed outside the hospital.

Medicare. The government's medical insurance program for people age 65 and older and for the disabled.

Medicare-approved amount. A dollar figure approved by Medicare that will be either the **usual and customary charge,** the prevailing charge, or the actual charge (whichever is lowest) and is the amount Medicare pays the doctor.

Medicare assignment. An agreement by a physician or medical provider to accept the Medicare-approved amount as payment in full for services rendered to a Medicare beneficiary.

Optionally renewable clause. A provision that gives an insurance company the right to cancel the coverage at any anniversary or, in some cases, at any premium due date. However, the company may not cancel the coverage between such dates.

Outpatient. Someone who receives services in a hospital but who is not admitted to the hospital.

Period of noncoverage. Provisions that specify periods when the insurance contract is not in force.

Policy. The legal document issued by the insurance company to you, the policyholder, that outlines the conditions and terms of the insurance. Also called the contract.

Policy limit. The maximum benefits an insurance company will pay under a particular policy.

Preexisting condition. A physical or mental condition that a person had before applying for insurance. Insurance companies often will not cover preexisting conditions.

Preferred provider organization (PPO). An organization of doctors and hospitals that provides medical services to groups of people at discounted rates. Members of the groups agree to use only the "preferred" providers.

Premium. The payment required to keep a policy active.

Prepaid plan. A plan that provides medical services to a group of persons who pay for the services in advance in the form of a monthly fee. Health maintenance organizations and individual practice associations are prepaid plans.

Rider. A document that amends the policy. It may increase or decrease benefits, waive the condition of coverage, or in any other way amend the original contract.

Schedule of benefits. A list of the maximum amounts payable for certain conditions.

Skilled nursing facility (SNF). A facility that provides skilled nursing care and related services for patients who require inpatient medical or nursing care.

Stop-loss provision. A provision that limits your out-of-pocket expenses to a set amount, after which the insurance policy pays all expenses up to the plan's maximum benefits.

Surgical schedule. A list of cash allowances that are payable for various types of surgery, with maximum allowances based upon the severity of the operation.

Third-party payer. An organization (such as an insurance company) that reimburses medical care providers (such as

hospitals and medical practitioners) for services provided
to policyholders.

Usual, customary, and reasonable. A charge for medical care
that is consistent with the going rate for identical or similar
services in the same geographic area.

Waiting period. The length of time an employee must wait from
his or her date of employment or application for insurance
coverage to the date his or her insurance goes into effect.

Worker's compensation insurance. An insurance program,
usually established by the state, that provides benefits to
employees who are injured in the course of their employment.

14

Medication Families

Drugs and medications are big business in the United States. Each year, Americans consume 16 tons of aspirin and fill approximately 200 million prescriptions for antibiotics. There are some 2,500 drugs on the market, and the number increases each year. Clearly, there's no way that consumers can become familiar with the names of all the available prescription and over-the-counter medications. But consumers can become acquainted with the basic types of medical drugs.

This section lists the basic families of medical drugs, highlights how they are used, and gives some examples. In the following examples, generic name comes first, and brand name follows in parentheses. As you read this section, be aware that *family* name is distinct from *generic* name. A drug family is a broad category that describes how a drug is used or what a drug is supposed to achieve; the generic name is more specific, referring to a certain chemical formula.

ACE inhibitor. Inhibits the body's ability to produce a chemical that causes arteries to tighten.

Analeptic. Stimulates the central nervous system. *Example:* methamphetamine (Desoxyn).

Analgesic. Relieves pain. *Examples:* aspirin, acetaminophen (Tylenol), ibuprofen (Motrin, Advil).

Anesthetic. Produces a loss of sensation. *Examples:* ether, procaine (Novocain), benzocaine.

Anorexiant. Suppresses the appetite. *Examples:* fenfluramine (Pondimin), dextroamphetamine (Dexedrine).

The Top 20 Prescription Drugs (1990)

1. Amoxil (antibiotic)
2. Lanoxin (cardiac)
3. Zantac (antiulcer)
4. Premarin (hormone)
5. Xanax (antianxiety)
6. Dyazide (diuretic/antihypertensive)
7. Cardizem (antiangina)
8. Synthroid (thyroid hormone)
9. Ceclor (antibiotic)
10. Seldane (antihistamine)
11. Vasotec (antihypertensive)
12. Tenormin (antihypertensive)
13. Procardia (antiangina)
14. Ortho-Novum 7/7/7 (oral contraceptive)
15. Capoten (antihypertensive)
16. Naprosyn (antiinflammatory)
17. Tagamet (antiulcer)
18. Calan (antiangina/antiarrythmia/antihypertensive)
19. Prozac (antidepressant)
20. Ortho-Novum (oral contraceptive)

Source: Pharmaceutical Data Services

Antacid. Neutralizes excess stomach acid. *Examples:* magnesium solution (Phillips Milk of Magnesia), magaldrate (Riopan), bicarbonate (Alka-Seltzer).

Anthelmintic. Destroys and expels intestinal worms. *Examples:* mebendazole (Vermox), thiabendazole (Mintezol).

Antiangina. Treats the symptoms of angina by widening the coronary arteries and reducing the work load on the heart. *Examples:* diltiazem (Cardizem), nifedipine (Procardia).

Antianxiety. Prevents and relieves fear and anxiety and relaxes muscles. *Examples:* alprazolam (Xanax), diazepam (Valium).

Antiarrhythmic. Controls heartbeat irregularities. *Examples:* verapamil (Calan, Isoptin), propranolol (Inderal).

Antiarthritic. Alleviates the symptoms of arthritis. *Examples:* aspirin (Ecotrin), piroxicam (Feldene).

Antiasthmatic. Treats asthma and related respiratory conditions. *Examples:* terbutaline (Brethine, Bricanyl), albuterol (Ventolin).

Antibacterial. Fights infection caused by bacteria. *Examples:* silver sulfadiazine (Flint SSD Cream), ampicillin, trimethoprim/sulfamethoxazole (Septra).

Antibiotic. Impedes or destroys the growth of microorganisms. *Examples:* penicillin, ampicillin, cephalosporin, tetracycline.

Anticaries agent. Protects teeth and bones against deterioration. *Example:* fluoride.

Anticholinergic. Decreases the actions of the respiratory, gastrointestinal, and urinary systems by blocking the action of acetylcholine, a chemical produced by the body. *Examples:* physostigmine salicylate (Antilirium), glycopyrrolate (Robinul).

Anticoagulant. Inhibits or prevents blood clotting. *Examples:* dicumarol (Dicumarol), heparin (Heparin).

Anticonvulsant. Prevents convulsions or epileptic seizures. *Examples:* phenytoin (Dilantin), ethotoin (Peganone), ethosuximide (Zarontin).

Antidepressant. Treats the symptoms of depression. *Examples:* amitriptyline (Elavil), doxepin (Adapin, Sinequan).

Antidiabetic. Assists in the treatment of diabetes. *Examples:* chlorpropamide (Diabinese), tolazamide (Tolinase).

Antidiarrheal. Relieves diarrhea. *Examples:* diphenoxylate (Lomotil), pectin/kaolin solution (Parepectolin).

Antiemetic. Relieves nausea and vomiting. *Examples:* dimenhydrinate (Dramamine), meclizine (Bonine, Antivert).

Antifungal. Kills or inhibits fungal organisms. *Examples:* nystatin (Mycostatin, Nilstat), clotrimazole (Lotrimin).

Antihistamine. Reduces or counteracts the effects of histamine, a chemical released during allergic reactions. *Examples:* diphenhydramine (Benadryl), chlorpheniramine (Comtrex).

Antihypertensive. Lowers blood pressure and treats arteriosclerosis (hardening of the arteries). *Examples:* atenolol (Tenormin), metoprolol (Lopressor).

Antiinfective. Combats infection.

Antiinflammatory. Reduces inflammation of tissue. *Examples:* aspirin, ibuprofen (Motrin), naproxen (Naprosyn), dexamethasone (Decadron).

Antinauseant. Suppresses nausea. *Examples:* dimenhydrinate (Dramamine), chlorpromazine (Thorazine).

Antineoplastic. Kills, damages, or restrains the growth of selected cells. Certain antibiotics, cytotoxic agents, and hormones are used as antineoplastics, among other drugs.

Antiparkinsonian. Treats Parkinson's disease. *Examples:* selegiline (Eldepryl), levodopa (Larodopa, Sinemet).

Antipruritic. Relieves itching. *Examples:* betamethasone dipropionate (Diprosone), clemastine fumarate (Tavist).

Antipyretic. Reduces fever. *Examples:* aspirin, acetaminophen (Tylenol).

Antiseptic. Inhibits the growth of microorganisms. *Example:* benzalkonium chloride (Mercurochrome II).

Antispasmodic. Reduces muscle spasms, particularly in the intestinal system. *Examples:* isopropamide iodide (Darbid), hyoscyamine sulfate (Levsin).

Antitoxin. Neutralizes poisonous microorganisms in the body. *Examples:* diphtheria antitoxin, tetanus antitoxin.

Antitussive. Suppresses coughing.

Antiulcer. Treats stomach ulcers. *Examples:* ranitidine (Zantac), cimetidine (Tagamet).

Astringent. Reduces swelling and bleeding by contracting blood vessels and tissues.

Beta-blocker. Slows the heartbeat and lowers blood pressure. *Examples:* propanolol (Inderal), metoprolol (Lopressor).

Bronchodilator. Widens the lung's air passages (bronchi). *Examples:* albuterol (Ventolin), theophylline (Aerolate, Theo-Dur).

Calcium channel blocker. Widens blood vessels and eases the work load on the heart. *Examples:* nimodipine (Nimotop), diltiazem (Cardizem).

Carbonic anhydrase inhibitor. Decreases pressure within the eye. *Example:* acetazolamide (Diamox).

Chelating agent. Removes unwanted minerals from the bloodstream. *Examples:* trientine (Cuprid), penicillamine (Depen).

Cholesterol reducer. Decreases the amount of cholesterol in the blood. *Examples:* dextrothyroxine (Choloxin), lovastatin (Mevacor).

Cholinergic. Increases the activity of the heart, lungs, and gastrointestinal tract and expands blood vessels.

Corticosteroid. Reduces inflammation and swelling or puffiness. *Examples:* cortisone, prednisone (Deltasone).

Cytotoxic. Kills or damages certain cells, such as cancer cells. See also **antineoplastic.** *Example:* tamoxifen (Nolvadex) for breast cancer.

Decongestant. Reduces swelling and congestion. *Example:* oxymetazoline (Afrin).

Demulcent. Soothes irritations of body surfaces.

Diaphoretic. Increases sweating.

Diuretic. Increases the amount of urine discharged by the body. *Examples:* furosemide (Lasix), chlorothiazide (Diuril).

Emetic. Induces vomiting. *Example:* ipecac syrup.

Expectorant. Stimulates coughing to clear mucus and phlegm from the throat and lungs. *Example:* guaifenesin (Robitussin).

Fibrinolytic. Dissolves newly formed blood clots in veins and arteries.

Hematinic. Increases the number of red blood cells in the blood. *Examples:* cyanocobalamin (Trinsicon), folic acid (Niferex).

Hormone. A chemical produced naturally by the body. Hormone extracts or synthetic hormones may be administered to counteract a hormone deficiency or, in the case of women on the Pill, to act as a method of contraception. *Examples:* estrogen and progesterone (female sex hormones), androsterone and testosterone (male sex hormones), insulin, adrenaline.

Hypnotic. Dulls the senses or induces sleep. *Examples:* sodium pentobarbital (Nembutal), ethchlorvynol (Placidyl).

Hypoglycemic. Lowers the level of sugar (glucose) in the blood. *Examples:* chlorpropamide (Diabinese), glyburide (DiaBeta, Micronase).

Immunosuppressant. Suppresses the immune system's tendency to attack diseases or foreign tissues introduced into the body. *Examples:* azathioprine (Imuran), cyclosporine.

Laxative. Stimulates bowel movements. *Examples:* mineral oil, psyllium preparations (Metamucil), phenolphthalein (Modane).

Muscle relaxant. Relieves muscle spasms or contractions. *Examples:* baclofen (Lioresal), methocarbamol (Robaxin).

Narcotic. Induces sleep, produces stupor, and relieves pain.

Psychotherapeutic. Treats emotional disorders.

Sedative. Calms and quiets the nerves. *Examples:* sodium pentobarbital (Nembutal), promethazine (Phenergan).

Thrombolytic. Dissolves blood clots. *Examples:* urokinase (Abbokinase), streptokinase (Streptase).

Tranquilizer. Reduces mental tension and anxiety. *Examples:* benzodiazepine (Limbitrol, Valium), phenothiazine (Thorazine).

Vasoconstrictor. Tightens (constricts) blood vessels. *Example:* norepinephrine (Levophed).

Vasodilator. Expands (dilates) blood vessels. *Examples:* isosorbide dinitrate (Isordil), minoxidil (Loniten).

CHAPTER

15

Measurements and Equivalents

If your doctor told you that you had a cyst two centimeters long, would you know precisely how large that cyst is? If your prescription said to take five milliliters of liquid medicine before each meal, would you know how much to pour? The medical system doesn't always function with the consumer's convenience in mind. Some of us are conversant in the metric system, while others prefer to have explanations given in the plain old American system of measurements. This chapter highlights metric measurements and gives you useful household equivalents.

Weights—Metric System
1 kilogram (kg)   = 1000 grams
1 gram (g, gm)   = 1000 milligrams
1 milligram (mg) = 1000 micrograms

Weight Equivalents (approximate)
65 milligrams   = 1 grain (gr)
28.35 grams   = 1 ounce (oz)
0.454 kilograms = 16 ounces (1 pound, or 1 lb)
   (454 grams)   (1 pound)
1 kilogram   = 2.2 pounds (lb)

Linear Measurement Equivalents (approximate)

1 millimeter (mm)	=	0.04 inch
1 centimeter (cm)	=	0.4 inch
2.5 centimeters	=	1 inch
30.5 centimeters	=	1 foot
1 meter	=	39.37 inches

Metric Liquid Measurements

1 liter (l)	=	1000 milliliters (ml) or
		100 centiliters (cl) or
		10 deciliters (dl)
1 deciliter (dl)	=	100 milliliters (ml) or
		10 centiliters (cl)
1 centiliter (cl)	=	10 milliliters (ml)

Liquid Measurement Equivalents (approximate)

4.7 milliliters	=	1 household teaspoonful
5 milliliters	=	1 medical teaspoonful
8 milliliters	=	1 dessertspoonful
15 milliliters	=	1 tablespoon (tbsp), 1/2 fluid ounce
30 milliliters	=	1 fluid ounce
60 milliliters	=	1 wineglassful
120 milliliters	=	1 teacupful
240 milliliters	=	8 fluid ounces, 1 cup
500 milliliters	=	1+ pint
1000 milliliters	=	1+ quart

Temperature Equivalents

Centigrade degrees		Fahrenheit degrees
0	Freezing	32
36.0		96.8
36.5		97.9
37.0		98.6
37.5		99.5
38.0		100.4

Temperature Equivalents, *continued*

Centigrade degrees		Fahrenheit degrees
38.5		101.3
39.0		102.2
39.5		103.1
40.0		104.0
40.5		104.9
41.0		105.8
100.0	Boiling	212.0

Temperature Conversion Formulas

To convert degrees Fahrenheit to degrees centigrade, subtract 32, then multiply by 0.555.

To convert degrees centigrade to degrees Fahrenheit, multiply by 1.8, then add 32.

ADDITIONAL READING

Current Medical Diagnosis and Treatment, 26th edition, by Marcus Krupp and Milton L. Chatton. Los Altos, CA: Appleton-Lange, 1987. A book for the consumer who wants to delve into a tome of medical information.

Dorland's Illustrated Medical Dictionary, 27th edition. Philadelphia: W. B. Saunders, 1988. The standard dictionary of medical terms written for medical professionals. Thorough, but often difficult to understand.

Medical Abbreviations: 7000 Conveniences at the Expense of Communications and Safety, by Neil M. Davis, M.S., Pharm.D. Huntington Valley, PA: Neil M. Davis Associates, 1990. All the medical abbreviations you'd need to know and then some. The author also explains how (and when) medical abbreviations endanger consumer health.

Medicare Made Easy, by Charles B. Inlander and Charles K. MacKay. Reading, MA: Addison-Wesley, 1992. A complete user's guide to the Medicare system, one of the most complex insurance programs of all.

Medication Guide for Patient Counseling, Dorothy L. Smith. Philadelphia: Lea and Febiger, 1981. The introductory chapters of this book are written for doctors, but the bulk of the text is an excellent chapter of medication instructions, written in language any consumer can understand.

Options in Health Care: Understanding Traditional and Alternative Methods. Allentown, PA: People's Medical Society, 1985. This booklet examines the many branches of the health care family tree, including traditional and mainstream modes of medical care as well as nontraditional and alternative health care systems.

The Patient's Guide to Medical Tests, 3rd and revised edition, by Cathey Pinckney and Edward R. Pinckney. New York: Facts on File, 1987. Information about hundreds of medical tests and their possible risks.

People's Book of Medical Tests, by David S. Sobel, M.D., and Tom Ferguson, M.D. New York: Summit Books, 1985. Down-to-earth and easy-to-understand discussions of approximately 200 medical tests and procedures.

Stedman's Abbrev.: Abbreviations, Acronyms & Symbols. Baltimore, MD: Williams & Wilkins, 1992.

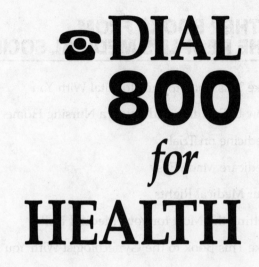

DIAL 800 *for* HEALTH

OTHER BOOKS FROM
THE PEOPLE'S MEDICAL SOCIETY

Take This Book to the Hospital With You

How to Evaluate and Select a Nursing Home

Medicine on Trial

Medicare Made Easy

Your Medical Rights

Getting the Most for Your Medical Dollar

Take This Book to the Gynecologist With You

Take This Book to the Obstetrician With You

Healthy Body Book: Test Yourself for Maximum Health

Blood Pressure: Questions You Have...Answers You Need

Your Heart: Questions You Have...Answers You Need

The Consumer's Guide to Medical Lingo

150 Ways to Be a Savvy Medical Consumer

100 Ways to Live to 100

Take This Book to the Pediatrician With You

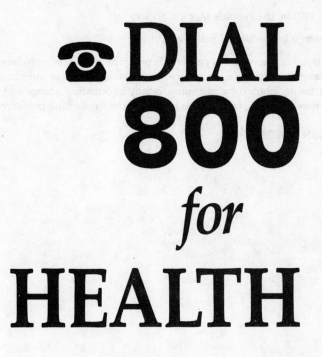

☎ DIAL 800

for

HEALTH

Compiled and Tested by the
People's Medical Society

≡ People's Medical Society
Allentown, Pennsylvania

ISBN 0-9627334-9-0

CONTENTS

Index and Subject Cross-Reference

INTRODUCTION

The emerging consumer health movement has spawned an army of well-informed, pro-active individuals who no longer limit their sources of health and medical information to their personal physicians. These empowered consumers now look to a wide array of professional and consumer-oriented organizations for vital medical and health care information. No longer do consumers have limited access to cutting-edge data about specific conditions, medications, or treatment options, to name just a few. A nationwide network of self-help and support groups has been formed around such interests as adoption services, organ transplants, substance abuse counseling, and women's health.

In this book, the People's Medical Society has assembled more than 300 useful and important health-related organizations that offer toll-free telephone numbers for public use. You are bound to find the right organization to help you in your specific search for necessary health data. For example, *Dial 800 for Health* gives you access to agencies and organizations that can tell you about a medical condition, answer your questions about toxic substances, test your hearing over the phone, or locate a local support group. And you don't need to leave your home to obtain any of this information. The only piece of equipment you need is your telephone.

With literally hundreds of groups to choose from, you're sure to find one that meets your particular needs and interests. And you won't spend a fortune making

long-distance calls. Some groups listed in this directory
are clearinghouses—services that can point you to an
organization in or near your own community to help you
directly. Others offer free information packets. Still others
have answering machines so you can leave your own
message or request additional information.

The majority of organizations listed in this book are
not-for-profit agencies, though a few are profit-making
businesses. Much of the information is provided free;
however, some organizations may charge a small service
fee for material they provide. In addition, these organizations may offer publications for sale. But rarely is there
a charge for the phone call.

The world of health is changing on a daily basis.
No single individual can keep up with all the new and
important information that emerges on a daily basis. But
Dial 800 for Health is your entree to vital medical and health
information that was previously hard to find.

Use it for good health.

HOW TO USE THIS DIRECTORY

Dial 800 for Health is like having your own personal health care researcher to provide you with answers and information you need to make important health care decisions. The table of contents alphabetically lists all major headings, such as adoption, cancer, health information, and orphan drugs. By turning directly to the pages listed for that particular heading, you will find the organizations and agencies that can help you. Included for each organization is the name, address, hours of operation, and the type of information or service provided. Many of these organizations are accessible to the hearing impaired and, where available, that number is also listed.

The index and subject cross-reference guide found in the back of the book can help you locate an agency or organization even if you can't find it listed in the table of contents. For example, if you want information on Crohn's disease and you don't find it listed among the major headings, you should turn to the alphabetical listings in the guide and locate Crohn's disease, which then directs you to look under "digestive diseases." Again, if you can't find a particular listing in the table of contents, then consult the index and subject cross-reference pages.

Types of Toll-Free Numbers

Most of the toll-free telephone numbers listed in this directory are accessible from every state. Just dial *1 + 800 + the number.* However, some organizations, such as the poison control centers, serve only one state or a limited portion of an adjoining state. When this is the case, we have listed the name of the state following the number, for example: 800-555-2345 *Colorado and Wyoming.*

Hours of operation are listed in local time zones, either eastern, central, mountain, or Pacific. All times shown are local, such as 8:00 a.m. to 6:00 p.m. Monday - Friday. There will be no reference to standard or daylight time.

Every toll-free number listed in this directory has been verified just prior to publication and found to be in operation. However, should you encounter a problem, we suggest you call the toll-free directory assistance operator at 800-555-1212.

A brief explanation follows the listing, which describes the type of service or information provided by the organization. This will help you determine if the organization does indeed provide the kind of information you desire.

The People's Medical Society makes no claims or guarantees for the organizations listed in this directory. *Dial 800 for Health* is not an endorsement or recommendation of these organizations by the People's Medical Society. We cannot be responsible for the services offered or the content of the information provided. As always, we encourage you to exercise your own good judgment when contacting any of these groups.

ADOPTION

AASK America
657 Mission Street, Suite 601
San Francisco, CA 94105
800-232-2751
> *Provides information on how to adopt children with special needs, such as mental and physical handicaps.*

Child Reach
155 Plan Way
Warwick, RI 02886
800-556-7918
> *Provides information on how to become a foster parent to Third World children.*

Concerned United Birthparents
2000 Walker Street
Des Moines, IA 50317
800-822-2777
515-263-9558 Iowa
> *Provides information on support groups designed for birthparents who gave up their child for adoption and are now seeking to come to terms with their decision. Makes referrals to support groups throughout the country.*

Edna Gladney Center
2300 Hemphill Street
Ft. Worth, TX 76110
800-433-2922
800-772-2740 Texas
8:30 a.m. to 5:00 p.m. (central time) Monday-Saturday
> *Provides counseling and shelter to single pregnant women who want to place their children for adoption. Free information packet available upon request.*

International Children's Care
2711 N.E. 134th Street
Vancouver, WA 98686
800-422-7729
> *Provides information to couples or individuals who are interested in foreign adoptions. Counsels prospective parents on the adoption and immigration laws of the foreign country.*

National Adoption Center
1218 Chestnut Street
Philadelphia, PA 19107
800-862-3678
215-925-0200 Philadelphia area
> *Provides adoption information concerning hard-to-place children and children with special needs.*

Pregnancy Counseling Services
Liberty Godparent Home
1000 Villa Road
Lynchburg, VA 24503
800-542-4453
804-384-3043 Virginia
24 hours a day
> *Provides information on residential programs for unwed mothers and offers counseling and adoption services. Also makes referrals to other support groups and similar homes in the caller's area.*

AEROBIC EXERCISE

Aerobic and Fitness Association of America
15250 Ventura Boulevard, Suite 310
Sherman Oaks, CA 91403
800-446-2322
800-445-5950
800-343-2584 California
800-225-2322 Canada and Mexico
8:30 a.m. to 5:00 p.m. (Pacific time) Monday-Friday
> *Provides basic information on aerobic exercise, certified instructors, and prevention and treatment of aerobics-related injuries.*

National Dance-Exercise Instructors Training Association
1503 South Washington Avenue, Suite 208
Minneapolis, MN 55454
800-237-6242
612-340-1306 Minnesota
> *Provides information on aerobics instructors and seminars nationwide.*

AIDS
(Acquired Immune Deficiency Syndrome)

AIDS Hotline
c/o American Social Health Association
P. O. Box 13827
Research Triangle Park, NC 27709
800-342-2437
800-243-7889 Hearing impaired
  24 hours a day
800-344-7432 Spanish
  8:00 a.m. to 2:00 a.m. (eastern time) 7 days a week
> *Provides information on HIV and AIDS transmission and prevention. Answers specific questions concerning HIV and AIDS and also makes referrals for testing and counseling. Free information packet available upon request.*

American Academy of Pediatrics
Pediatric AIDS Coalition
1331 Pennsylvania Avenue, N.W., Suite 721-N
Washington, DC 20004
800-336-5475
202-662-7460 District of Columbia
9:00 a.m. to 5:00 p.m. (eastern time) Monday-Friday
Provides information on AIDS-education programs for adults and children in churches, schools, and other community organizations.

Clinical Trials Information Service
P. O. Box 6421
Rockville, MD 20849-6421
800-874-2572
800-243-7012 Hearing impaired
9:00 a.m. to 7:00 p.m. (eastern time) Monday-Friday
Provides information on the status of federally and privately sponsored experimental drug trials for HIV and AIDS. Free materials available upon request.

Haitian AIDS Hotline
8037 N.E. Second Avenue
Miami, FL 33138
800-722-7432
8:30 a.m. to 5:00 p.m. (eastern time) Monday-Friday
Provides HIV and AIDS information specifically tailored to the Haitian population.

Multicultural Training Resource Center
1540 Market Street, Suite 320
San Francisco, CA 94102
800-545-6642 California
Provides HIV and AIDS information specifically targeted to diverse cultural groups.

Names Project
2362 Market Street
P. O. Box 14573
San Francisco, CA 94114
800-872-6263 California
415-863-5511
9:00 a.m. to 6:00 p.m. (Pacific time) Monday-Friday
Provides information on how to add names to the AIDS Memorial Quilt project, which commemorates those men, women, and children who have lost their lives to AIDS.

National AIDS Information Clearinghouse
P. O. Box 6003
Rockville, MD 20849-6003
800-458-5231
9:00 a.m. to 7:00 p.m. (eastern time) Monday-Friday
*Provides recorded messages in English and Spanish with information
on organizational and educational materials, clinical drug trials, and
how to order publications.*

National Association of People With AIDS
2025 I Street, N.W., Suite 1118
Washington, DC 20006
800-673-8538
*Provides information and referrals to local chapters of People With AIDS.
Also maintains a national system of self-empowering programs for
people infected with HIV or who have AIDS-Related Complex or AIDS.*

National Native American AIDS Prevention Center
3515 Grand Avenue, Suite 100
Oakland, CA 94610
800-283-2437
8:30 a.m. to 5:00 p.m. (Pacific time) Monday-Friday
510-444-2051 Oakland area
510-444-1593 FAX
*Provides referrals to counseling and testing centers. Free information
packet available upon request.*

Project Inform
220 Market Street
San Francisco, CA 94103
800-822-7422
800-334-7422 California
10:00 a.m. to 4:00 p.m. (Pacific time) Monday-Friday
10:00 a.m. to 1:00 p.m. (Pacific time) Saturday
Answering machine at all other times
*Provides current information on treatment options for persons with
HIV and AIDS, as well as information on organizations that provide
the treatments. Also operates an outreach and advocacy program.*

Teens Teaching AIDS Prevention
3030 Walnut Street
Kansas City, MO 64108
800-234-8336
816-561-8784 Kansas City area
4:00 p.m. to 8:00 p.m. (central time) Monday-Friday
Answering machine at all other times
*Provides information and counseling on HIV and AIDS from a teen's
perspective. Makes referrals to AIDS organizations and other resources.
Some literature available at a nominal charge.*

ALLERGIES AND ASTHMA

Allergy Information Referral Line
American Academy of Allergy and Immunology
611 East Wells Street
Milwaukee, WI 53202
800-822-2762
414-272-6071 Wisconsin
8:00 a.m to 5:00 p.m. (central time) Monday-Friday
> *Provides information on the diagnosis and treatment of allergies and asthma and makes referrals to allergy specialists.*

American College of Allergy and Immunology
800 West Northwest Highway, Suite 1080
Palatine, IL 60067
800-842-7777
24 hours a day, Monday-Friday
> *Provides information on various allergies and the treatment options available.*

Asthma and Allergy Foundation of America
1717 Massachusetts Avenue, N.W., Suite 305
Washington, DC 20036
800-727-8462
202-466-7643 District of Columbia
> *Provides U.S. maps showing zones where plants are likely to cause allergic problems. Also provides educational materials on asthma and allergies.*

National Jewish Asthma Center
1400 Jackson Street
Denver, CO 80206
800-222-5864
303-398-1477 Denver
8:00 a.m. to 5:00 p.m. (mountain time) Monday-Friday
> *Answers questions about asthma, emphysema, chronic bronchitis, and other respiratory diseases. Also makes referrals to doctors in caller's local area. Free information packets available upon request.*

ALZHEIMER'S DISEASE

Alzheimer's Association
919 North Michigan Avenue, Suite 1000
Chicago, IL 60611
800-272-3900
8:30 a.m. to 5:00 p.m. (central time) Monday-Friday
Answering machine at all other times
> *Provides information on Alzheimer's and related disorders and also makes referrals to local chapters of the association.*

American Health Assistance Foundation
15825 Shady Grove Road, Suite 140
Rockville, MD 20850
800-437-2423
301-948-3244 Maryland
9:00 a.m. to 5:00 p.m. (eastern time) Monday-Friday
*Provides public education materials on Alzheimer's relief programs
and provides funding for such programs. Also provides financial
assistance to families in need of relief services.*

AMYOTROPHIC LATERAL SCLEROSIS
(ALS) ("Lou Gehrig's Disease")

ALS Association
21021 Ventura Boulevard, Suite 321
Woodland Hills, CA 91364
800-782-4747
818-340-7500 San Fernando Valley
8:00 a.m. to 5:00 p.m. (Pacific time) Monday-Friday
*Provides education, information, and referral services to ALS patients
and their families. Also makes referrals to local chapters and
support groups.*

ANEMIA

Cooley's Anemia Foundation
105 East 22nd Street, Room 911
New York, NY 10010
800-221-3571
800-522-7222 New York
9:00 a.m. to 5:00 p.m. (eastern time) Monday-Friday
*Provides information on patient care, support groups, and the latest
research into Cooley's anemia.*

National Association for Sickle Cell Disease
3345 Wilshire Boulevard, Suite 1106
Los Angeles, CA 90010-1880
800-421-8453
213-736-5455 Los Angeles
8:30 a.m. to 5:00 p.m. (Pacific time) Monday-Friday
*Provides materials, trains counselors, and offers programs to medical
professionals and the public. Also supports research, conducts public
education campaigns, and provides diagnostic screening.*

ARTHRITIS

Arthritis Consulting Services
4620 North State Road 7, Suite 206
Ft. Lauderdale, FL 33319
800-327-3027
8:30 a.m. to 4:00 p.m. (eastern time) Monday-Friday
Provides information on holistic approaches to treating arthritis.

Arthritis Foundation Information Line
P. O. Box 19000
Atlanta, GA 30326
800-283-7800
404-872-7100 Georgia
9:00 a.m. to 7:00 p.m. (eastern time) Monday-Friday
Provides local physician referrals and information concerning local chapters of the Arthritis Foundation. Free brochures and other literature available upon request.

BLOOD DISORDERS

National Marrow Donor Program
3433 Broadway Street, N.E., Suite 400
Minneapolis, MN 55413-1762
800-654-1247
8:00 a.m. to 5:00 p.m. (central time) Monday-Friday
Answering machine at all other times
Maintains a registry of bone marrow donors and also provides information on how interested individuals can become active in the registry program.

BURN CARE

Phoenix Society
National Organization for Burn Survivors
11 Rust Hill Road
Levittown, PA 19056
800-888-2876
215-946-BURN
Provides information on the self-help services available to burn victims and their families. Helps burn victims deal with their trauma and provides the psychological support they need to return to normal lives and interests. Distributes information on burns and trauma and their treatment.

Shriners Hospital Referral Line
2900 Rocky Point Drive
Tampa, FL 33607-1435
800-237-5055
800-282-9161 Florida
8:00 a.m. to 5:00 p.m. (eastern time) Monday-Friday
Provides information about burn treatment programs available at Shriners hospitals.

CANCER

American Association of Oral and Maxillofacial Surgeons
9700 Bryn Mawr Avenue
Rosemont, IL 60018
800-467-5268
8:30 a.m. to 5:00 p.m. (central time) Monday-Friday
Answering machine at all other times
Provides information on oral cancer and makes referrals to oral surgeons in the caller's area.

American Cancer Society
1599 Clifton Road N.E.
Atlanta, GA 30329
800-227-2345
8:30 a.m. to 4:30 p.m. (eastern time) Monday-Friday
Provides general information on the society's programs and services and makes referrals to local chapters. Also answers questions about cancer, including prevention, diagnosis, treatment, and rehabilitation.

American Institute for Cancer Research
Nutrition Hotline
1759 R Street, N.W.
Washington, DC 20009
800-843-8114
202-328-7744 District of Columbia
9:00 a.m. to 9:00 p.m. (eastern time) Monday-Thursday
9:00 a.m. to 5:00 p.m. (eastern time) Friday
Answering machine at all other times
Provides information on the role of diet and nutrition in cancer prevention and how nutrition may be used to assist a cancer treatment program. Also responds to specific requests.

American Medical Center
Cancer Information and Counseling Line
1600 Pierce Street
Denver, CO 80214
800-525-3777
303-233-6501 Denver area
8:30 a.m. to 4:45 p.m. (mountain time) Monday-Friday
Provides the latest information on cancer prevention, detection and
treatment methods. Also offers counseling and makes referrals to
support groups.

Breast Cancer Hotline
Physicians Committee for Responsible Medicine
P. O. Box 6322
Washington, DC 20015
800-875-4837
9:00 a.m. to 5:00 p.m. (eastern time) Monday-Friday
Answering machine at all other times
Provides information on the link between diet and breast cancer.
Caller may leave name and address to receive a free packet
of information.

Candlelighters Childhood Cancer Foundation
7910 Woodmont Avenue, Suite 460
Bethesda, MD 20814
800-366-2223
24 hours a day
Provides information and services, such as a 24-hour crisis line and
transportation, to families of childhood cancer patients. Serves as a
clearinghouse and liaison between parents and medical professionals.
Established Ronald McDonald houses where family members of
patients may stay while the patient undergoes treatment.

Midwestern Regional Medical Center
2501 Emmaus Avenue
Zion, IL 60099
800-FOR-HELP
708-872-4561
Provides information on cancer treatment programs available at
the hospital.

National Cancer Institute
Cancer Information Service
9000 Rockville Pike, Suite 414
Bethesda, MD 20892
800-422-6237
800-638-6070 Alaska
800-524-1234 Hawaii
9:00 a.m. to 10:00 p.m. (eastern time) Monday-Friday
Provides information on various types of cancers and the latest
treatments available for those cancers. Free information is available
in both English and Spanish.

Y-Me Breast Cancer Support Program
18220 Harwood Avenue
Homewood, IL 60430
800-221-2141
708-799-8228 Illinois
> Provides information and support to women undergoing treatment for breast cancer. Also provides information on prostheses after breast surgery.

CEREBRAL PALSY

United Cerebral Palsy Association
7 Penn Plaza, Suite 804
New York, NY 10001
800-872-1827
212-268-6655 New York City area
9:00 a.m. to 5:00 p.m. (eastern time) Monday-Friday
> Provides information on the diagnosis and treatment of cerebral palsy and works to establish local programs that help people with the disease move into mainstream society.

CHILDREN'S SERVICES

American Academy of Pediatrics
P. O. Box 927
141 N.W. Point Boulevard
Elk Grove, IL 60007
800-433-9016
800-421-0589 Illinois
> Provides information on pediatric care and the role of the pediatrician.

American Association for Protecting Children
Division of American Humane Association
63 Inverness Drive East
Englewood, CO 80112
800-227-5242
303-792-9900 Colorado
8:30 a.m. to 5:00 p.m. (mountain time) Monday-Friday
Answering machine at all other times
> Provides services to professionals who work in the child-protection field and conducts research and program evaluations of child welfare agencies. List of books and other publications available upon request.

Boystown Hotline
Father Flanagan's Boystown
Boystown, NE 68010
800-448-3000
> *Provides assistance to runaway and homeless children regardless of race, color, or creed.*

Child Find
P. O. Box 277
New Paltz, NY 12561
800-426-5678
914-255-1848 New York
> *Operates an international locator service for missing children and maintains a registry of missing children.*

Children's Defense Fund
122 C Street, N.W., Suite 400
Washington, DC 20001
800-CDF-1200
202-628-8787 District of Columbia
> *Provides information on the expanding field of children's rights as recognized by law and is involved in social and educational programs affecting children. Free information available upon request.*

Children's Wish Foundation
7840 Roswell Road, Suite 301
Atlanta, GA 30350
800-323-9474
404-393-9474 Georgia
> *Provides information on programs that seek to grant a dying child his or her final wish. Works with organizations and individuals who want to become Wish Foundation supporters.*

Covenant House
460 West 41st Street
New York, NY 10036
800-999-9999
> *Provides 24-hour assistance to runaways and homeless youth. Also provides temporary shelter until the child's situation at home can be resolved.*

Feingold Association of the United States
P. O. Box 6550
Alexandria, VA 22306
800-321-3287
24 hours a day
> *Provides information on the Feingold Program, which uses diet to treat children with learning and behavioral problems. Also makes referrals to local support groups. Free information available upon request.*

"Just Say No" Kids Club International
2101 Webster Street, Suite 1300
Oakland, CA 94612
800-258-2766
510-939-6666

> *Provides information on drug prevention programs for children and on how to start a "Just Say No" chapter.*

Kevin Collins Foundation for Missing Children
P. O. Box 590473
San Francisco, CA 94159
800-272-0012

> *Provides counseling and education to families of missing or abducted children and helps them through the ordeal.*

Kidsrights
10100 Park Cedar Drive
Charlotte, NC 28210
800-892-5437

> *Provides information to parents and other interested individuals on how to establish programs that work to combat teen suicide.*

Missing Children Awareness Foundation
13094 95th Street North
Largo, FL 34643
800-741-7233

> *Provides assistance and referrals to parents of missing children.*

Missing Children Help Center
410 Ware Boulevard, Suite 400
Tampa, FL 33619
800-872-5437

> *Provides assistance to parents of missing children by publicizing the children's photographs in newspapers, brochures, and flyers.*

National Association for the Education of Young Children
1834 Connecticut Avenue, N.W.
Washington, DC 20009
800-424-2460

> *Provides information and referrals to accredited child-care programs.*

National Child Watch Campaign
P. O. Box 1368
Jackson, MI 49204
800-222-1464

> *Provides information on child safety and how to establish a child-watch program to protect children from being kidnapped. Also provides counseling and support services to parents whose child has been kidnapped or is missing.*

National Hotline for Missing and Exploited Children
2101 Wilson Boulevard, Suite 550
Arlington, VA 22201
800-843-5678
7:30 a.m. to 11:00 p.m. (eastern time) Monday-Friday
10:00 a.m. to 6:00 p.m. (eastern time) Saturday
Operates a hotline for reporting sightings of missing children and children exploited by crime, prostitution, and pornography. Provides technical assistance to legal authorities in the hunt for missing or kidnapped children.

National Information Clearinghouse for Infants With Disabilities and Life-Threatening Conditions
University of South Carolina
Benson Building, 1st Floor
Columbia, SC 29208
800-922-9234 Voice- and hearing-impaired
800-922-1107 Voice- and hearing-impaired (South Carolina)
9:00 a.m.. to 5:00 p.m. (eastern time) Monday-Friday
Answering machine at all other times
Provides information to families with children who have rare or life-threatening conditions. Also offers referrals to professional and community services in the caller's area. Offers special services to Vietnam veterans and their families.

National Resource Center on Child Sexual Abuse
107 Lincoln Street
Huntsville, AL 35801
800-543-7006
Provides resources to agencies dealing with children who have been sexually abused. Also provides bibliographies and articles on the sexual abuse of children.

National Runaway Hotline
Office of the Governor
P. O. Box 12428
Austin, TX 78711
800-231-6946
800-392-3352 Texas
Provides assistance to runaway children by making referrals to shelters and other agencies. Also delivers messages to the families of runaway children.

National Runaway Switchboard
3080 North Lincoln
Chicago, IL 60657
800-621-4000
Provides counseling and referral to runaway youths 18 years of age and younger.

Operation Lookout National Center for Missing Youth
P. O. Box 231
Mount Lake Terrace, WA 98043
800-782-7335
> *Provides assistance in locating missing children.*

Parent Help Line
Nashua Brookside Hospital
11 Northwest Boulevard
Nashua, NH 03063
800-543-6381
> *Provides referrals to organizations that can aid parents in obtaining treatment and counseling for troubled kids.*

Shriners Hospital Referral Line
2900 Rocky Point Drive
Tampa, FL 33607-1435
800-237-5055
800-282-9161 Florida
8:00 a.m. to 5:00 p.m. (eastern time) Monday-Friday
> *Provides information about children's services available at Shriners hospitals.*

Teen Crisis Hotline
498 South Spring Street
Crestview, FL 32536
800-262-8336 Florida
> *Provides information and referrals to teenagers facing crises in their lives.*

Toughlove International
P. O. Box 1069
Doylestown, PA 18901
800-333-1069
215-348-7090 Pennsylvania
> *Serves as a support group for parents of children with behavioral problems. Makes referrals in both the United States and Canada.*

Vanished Children's Alliance
1407 Parkmoor Avenue, Suite 200
San Jose, CA 95126
800-826-4743
408-971-4822
24 hours a day
> *Provides information on missing and recovered children.*

Youth Crisis Hotline
10225 Ulmerton Road, Suite 4-A
Largo, FL 34641
800-442-4673
> *Provides information on child abuse and serves as an advocacy group for abused children.*

CLEFT PALATE

American Cleft Palate Educational Foundation
1218 Grandview Avenue
Pittsburgh, PA 15211
800-24-CLEFT
800-242-5338
800-232-5338 Pennsylvania
Assists parents by providing information about feeding, dental care, and local professionals and support groups. Free information available upon request.

CORNELIA DE LANGE SYNDROME (CDLS)

Cornelia de Lange Foundation
60 Dyer Avenue
Collinsville, CT 06022
800-223-8355
800-753-2357 Canada
9:00 a.m. to 4:30 p.m. (eastern time) Monday-Friday
Answering machine at all other times
Provides general information on the birth defects caused by CDLS. Operates a support system for parents and makes referrals to local chapters. Free information available upon request.

DENTAL CARE

American Academy of Cosmetic Dentistry
2711 Marshall Court
Madison, WI 53705
800-543-9220
Provides information on cosmetic dentistry and referrals to practitioners in the caller's area.

American Association of Orthodontists
460 North Lindbergh Boulevard
St. Louis, MO 63141
800-222-9969
Provides information on orthodontic treatments and referrals to orthodontists in the caller's area.

Environmental Dental Association
9974 Scripps Ranch Boulevard, Suite 36
San Diego, CA 92131
800-388-8124
> *Provides information on alternatives to mercury fillings and how to locate dentists who do not use mercury fillings.*

DIABETES MELLITUS

American Diabetes Association
1660 Duke Street
Alexandria, VA 22314
800-232-3472
703-549-1500
8:30 a.m. to 5:00 p.m. (eastern time) Monday-Friday
> *Provides general information on the diagnosis and treatment of diabetes. Information packets available upon request.*

Diabetes Center, Inc.
P. O. Box 47945
Minneapolis, MN 55447
800-848-2793
> *Provides information on diabetic supplies, including prescription medications.*

Juvenile Diabetes Foundation
432 Park Avenue South
New York, NY 10016
800-223-1138
212-889-7575
> *Provides information on the latest research into the cause and prevention of juvenile diabetes. Also provides grants to support ongoing research.*

DIGESTIVE DISEASES

Crohn's and Colitis Foundation
444 Park Avenue South
New York, NY 10018
800-343-3637
9:00 a.m. to 5:00 p.m. (eastern time) Monday-Friday
> *Provides information on digestive diseases and their diagnosis and treatment. Also makes referrals to support groups and local chapters of the organization. Free literature available upon request.*

DOMESTIC VIOLENCE

Hit Home Youth Crisis Line
Youth Development International
P. O. Box 178408
San Diego, CA 92177-8408
800-448-4663
619-292-5683
> *Provides counseling and referrals on child abuse, runaways, suicide, molestation, and pregnancy.*

National Child Abuse Hotline
ChildHelp USA
P. O. Box 630
Hollywood, CA 90028
800-422-4453
24 hours a day
> *Provides 24-hour crisis counseling and intervention for any abuse-related situation. Also offers information and referral service that includes national, regional, or local organizations, agencies, and groups. Free literature available upon request.*

National Council on Child Abuse and Family Violence
1155 Connecticut Avenue, N.W., Suite 300
Washington, DC 20036
800-222-2000
202-429-6695 District of Columbia
7:30 a.m. to 4:30 p.m. (eastern time) Monday-Friday
> *Provides referrals to local community services and support groups. Free information packet available upon request.*

Parents Anonymous/Abusive Parents
520 South Lafayette Park Place, Suite 316
Los Angeles, CA 90057
800-421-0353
800-352-0386 California
8:30 a.m. to 5:00 p.m. (Pacific time) Monday-Friday
Answering machine at all other times
> *Provides information on the prevention and treatment of child abuse. Also makes referrals to self-help groups and local chapters for parents involved in abusive situations.*

DOWN SYNDROME

National Down Syndrome Congress
1800 Dempster Street
Park Ridge, IL 60068
800-232-6372
9:00 a.m. to 5:00 p.m. (central time) Monday-Friday
> *Provides information and referrals for families concerning Down
> syndrome. Publishes a newsletter and sponsors an annual convention.*

National Down Syndrome Society
666 Broadway
New York, NY 10012
800-221-4602
9:00 a.m. to 5:00 p.m. (eastern time) Monday-Friday
Answering machine at all other times
> *Provides free information packets on Down syndrome and makes
> referrals to local support groups in caller's area. Publications available
> for a small fee.*

DRINKING WATER

GEO/Resource Consultant, Inc.
1555 Wilson Boulevard, Suite 500
Arlington, VA 22209
800-426-4791
8:00 a.m. to 5:00 p.m. (eastern time) Monday-Friday
> *Provides information on drinking water standards that must be met
> by community and municipal water supplies.*

DRUG AND ALCOHOL
TREATMENT PROGRAMS

See: **SUBSTANCE ABUSE**

DYSLEXIA

Orton Dyslexia Society
Chester Building, Suite 382
8600 LaSalle Road
Baltimore, MD 21286-2044
800-222-3123
410-296-0232 Baltimore
9:00 a.m. to 5:00 p.m. (eastern time) Monday-Friday
> *Provides information on support networks and resources for people
> with dyslexia.*

EATING DISORDERS

FIT-AHL
Food Addiction Hotline
2000 Commerce Street
Melbourne, FL 32904
800-872-0088
> *Provides information on eating disorders and makes referrals to local services. Information packets available upon request.*

Take Off Pounds Sensibly (TOPS)
4575 South 5th Street
Milwaukee, WI 53207
800-932-8677
> *Provides information on sensible dieting methods. Also makes referrals to local chapters of TOPS.*

EMERGENCY MEDICAL COMMUNICATION SYSTEMS

American Medical Alert Corporation
3265 Lawson Boulevard
Oceanside, NY 11572
800-645-3244
> *Provides information on telecommunication devices that are used by people with life-threatening conditions or, in the case of accidents, that can be used to summon help in emergency situations.*

Lifeline Systems
1 Arsenal Marketplace
Watertown, MA 02172
800-451-0525
617-923-4141 Alaska, Hawaii, and Massachusetts
> *Provides information on communication systems that link elderly and handicapped persons directly to hospitals.*

ENDOMETRIOSIS

Endometriosis Association
8585 North 76th Place
Milwaukee, WI 53223
800-992-3636
800-426-2363 Canada
24 hours a day
> *Provides free information on endometriosis.*

EPILEPSY

Epilepsy Foundation of America
4351 Garden City Drive
Landover, MD 20785
800-332-1000
9:00 a.m. to 6:00 p.m. (eastern time) Monday-Friday
Provides information on the diagnosis and treatment of epilepsy and makes referrals to doctors in caller's area. Also operates a discount pharmacy available to members.

HANDICAPPED SERVICES

American Paralysis Association
500 Morris Avenue
Springfield, NJ 07081
800-225-0292
800-526-3456 New Jersey
8:30 a.m. to 5:00 p.m. (eastern time) Monday-Friday
Provides information on the treatment of spinal cord injuries and makes referrals to local support groups. Free information packet available upon request.

AT&T National Special Needs Center
2001 Route 46, Suite 310
Parsippany, NJ 07054
800-233-1222
800-833-3232 Hearing impaired
8:30 a.m. to 7:00 p.m. (eastern time) Monday-Friday
Provides information on special equipment available to people with hearing, speech, vision, or motion impairment.

Devereux Foundation
19 South Waterloo Road
Devon, PA 19333
800-345-1292 (Ext. 3109)
8:45 a.m. to 9:00 p.m. (eastern time) Monday-Friday
Provides information on treatment programs for children, adolescents, and adults with psychiatric, emotional, neurological, and developmental handicaps.

IBM National Support Center for People With Disabilities
P. O. Box 2150
Atlanta, GA 30301
800-426-2133
Provides information on how computers can assist the disabled.

Institute of Logopedics
2400 Jardine Drive
Wichita, KS 67219
800-835-1043
800-937-4644 (Includes Canada)
8:00 a.m. to 5:00 p.m. (central time) Monday-Friday
Provides information on residential programs for children with multiple disabilities.

Job Accommodation Network
809 Allen Hall
P. O. Box 6123
West Virginia University
Morgantown, WV 26506-6123
800-526-7234
800-526-4698 West Virginia
Provides information to employers and the public on how to accommodate the disabled in the workplace.

National Association of Rehabilitation Facilities
P. O. Box 17675
Washington, DC 20041
800-368-3513
8:30 a.m. to 5:30 p.m. (eastern time) Monday-Friday
Answering machine at all other times
Provides the names and locations of rehabilitation facilities. Also makes referrals to local support groups.

National Center for Youth With Disabilities
University of Minnesota Box 721
420 Delaware Street N.E.
Minneapolis, MN 55455
800-333-6293
612-624-3939 Hearing impaired
7:45 a.m. to 4:30 p.m. (central time) Monday-Friday
Provides free information to assist parents, educators, caregivers, advocates, and others in helping children and youth with disabilities become fully participating members of society.

National Clearinghouse on Postsecondary Education for Individuals With Disabilities
One Dupont Circle, Suite 800
Washington, DC 20036-1193
800-544-3284
202-939-9320 District of Columbia
Provides information for disabled individuals on job opportunities following graduation from high school.

National Easter Seal Society
70 East Lake Street
Chicago, IL 60601
800-221-6827
8:30 a.m. to 5:00 p.m. (central time) Monday-Friday
> *Provides information on therapy, counseling and educational programs for the disabled. Also makes referrals to community-based programs operated by the Easter Seal Society.*

National Information Center for Children and Youth With Disabilities
7926 Jones Branch Drive
McLean, VA 22102
800-999-5599
703-893-6061 Virginia
> *Provides information on programs for handicapped children and youth.*

National Organization on Disability
910 16th Street, N.W., Suite 600
Washington, DC 20006
800-248-2253
> *Provides information on how to improve living conditions for disabled individuals.*

National Rehabilitation Information Center
8455 Colesville Road, Suite 935
Silver Spring, MD 20910-3319
800-346-2742
8:00 a.m. to 6:00 p.m. (eastern time) Monday-Friday
> *Provides information on research, resources, and products for the disabled.*

National Tour Association
Handicapped Travel Division
546 East Main Street
Lexington, KY 40508
800-682-8886
> *Provides information to travelers who require special accommodations because of handicaps or other limitations. Provides a list of travel operators who have booked accommodations for handicapped individuals.*

Pathways Awareness Foundation
123 North Wacker Drive
Chicago, IL 60606
800-955-2445
9:00 a.m. to 5:00 p.m. (central time) Monday-Friday
> *Provides information on the detection of disabilities in early childhood.*

Tele-Consumer Hotline
1910 K Street, N.W., Suite 610
Washington, DC 20006
800-332-1124
Assists the disabled in locating communications equipment that can be adapted to their individual needs.

HANSON'S DISEASE
(Leprosy)

American Leprosy Missions
One American Leprosy Mission Way
Greenville, SC 29601
800-543-3131
8:00 a.m. to 5:00 p.m. (eastern time) Monday-Friday
Provides information on the diagnosis and treatment of Hanson's disease and makes referrals to treatment programs. Free information packet available upon request.

HEAD INJURY

National Head Injury Foundation
1776 Massachusetts Avenue, N.W., Suite 100
Washington, DC 20036
800-444-6443
202-296-6443 District of Columbia
9:00 a.m. to 5:00 p.m. (eastern time) Monday-Friday
Provides information on the treatment of head injuries and makes referrals to local support groups.

HEADACHE

National Headache Foundation
5252 North Western Avenue
Chicago, IL 60625
800-843-2256
9:00 a.m. to 5:00 p.m. (central time) Monday-Friday
Provides general information on the diagnosis and treatment of headaches. Also makes referrals to local support and mutual aid groups.

New England Headache Treatment Program
778 Longridge Road
Stamford, CT 06902
800-245-0088
203-968-1799 Connecticut
9:00 a.m. to 4:00 p.m. (eastern time) Monday-Friday
> *Provides general information on headaches and treatment programs available at Greenwich Hospital in Greenwich, Connecticut. Free information available upon request.*

HEALTH INFORMATION

American Institute for Preventive Medicine
30445 Northwestern Highway
Farmington Hills, MI 48075
800-345-2476
313-539-1800 Michigan
8:30 a.m. to 5:30 p.m. (eastern time) Monday-Friday
> *Provides information on programs designed for lifestyle improvement, such as stress reduction, weight control, smoking cessation, and health education. Free information available upon request.*

American Medical Radio News
515 North State Street
Chicago, IL 60610
800-448-9384
> *Provides a recorded message on a current health topic or feature story in medicine.*

American Osteopathic Association
142 East Ontario Street
Chicago, IL 60611
800-621-1773
312-280-5800
8:30 a.m. to 4:30 p.m. (central time) Monday-Friday
> *Provides information on osteopathic medicine and makes referrals to local osteopathic physicians and medical centers.*

American Trauma Society
8903 Presidential Parkway, Suite 512
Upper Marlboro, MD 20772-2656
800-556-7890
301-420-4189
9:00 a.m. to 5:00 p.m. (eastern time) Monday-Friday
> *Provides information on injury prevention and trauma care. Free information available upon request.*

California Self-Help Center
UCLA Psychology Department
405 Hilgard Avenue
Los Angeles, CA 90024
800-222-5465 California
> *Provides consumer information on a variety of health topics and makes*
> *referrals to local, regional, and national organizations.*

Center for Self Help
Riverwood Center
P. O. Box 547
Benton Harbor, MI 49022-0547
800-336-0341 Michigan
> *Provides information on self-help resources available in the*
> *caller's area.*

Consumer Health Information Resource Institute
3521 Broadway
Kansas City, MO 64111
800-821-6671
816-753-8850
9:00 a.m. to 5:00 p.m. (central time) Monday-Friday
> *Provides referrals to local, regional, and national organizations and*
> *also maintains a patient education library. Suggests sources of health*
> *information on various conditions, procedures, and medications.*

Doctor Referral Service of Mt. Sinai Medical Center
1 Gustave L. Levy Place
P. O. Box 1083
New York, NY 10029-6575
800-637-4624
8:30 a.m. to 6:00 p.m. (eastern time) Monday-Friday
> *Provides referrals to physicians located in the New York City area who*
> *are affiliated with Mt. Sinai Medical Center.*

Health Information Network International
4213 Montgomery Drive
Santa Rosa, CA 95405
800-743-6996
707-539-3967
9:00 a.m. to 5:00 p.m. (Pacific time) Monday-Friday
> *Provides consumers with the latest research and information on*
> *natural health substances, medical conditions, and treatment*
> *alternatives.*

Joseph and Rose Kennedy Institute of Ethics
National Reference Center for Bioethics Literature
Georgetown University
Washington, DC 20057
800-633-3849
202-687-3885

> *Provides information to medical professionals and the public on the topic of medical bioethics.*

National Health Information Center
U.S. Department of Health and Human Services
Office of Disease Prevention and Health Promotion
P. O. Box 1133
Washington, DC 20013
800-336-4797
301-565-4167 Maryland
9:00 a.m. to 5:00 p.m. (eastern time) Monday-Friday

> *Provides information to consumers and professionals on a variety of health-related topics. Also makes referrals to national organizations. Free literature available upon request.*

National Library of Medicine
8600 Rockville Pike, 4th Floor
Bethesda, MD 20894
800-638-8480

> *Provides computer access to medical literature and information-retrieval systems. Also searches current medical literature on a variety of topics.*

New Jersey Self-Help Clearinghouse
St. Clares-Riverside Hospital
Denville, NJ 07834
800-367-6274 New Jersey
201-625-7101
201-625-9053 Hearing impaired

> *Provides information to consumers on self-help groups and other organizations. Produces materials on how to establish a self-help group. Also publishes a directory of self-help and mutual aid organizations.*

Office of Minority Health
Resource Center
1010 Wayne Avenue, Suite 300
Silver Spring, MD 20910
800-444-6472
9:00 a.m. to 5:00 p.m. (eastern time) Monday-Friday

> *Provides information to minority groups on health topics that are of special interest to them. Free information packet available upon request. English and Spanish language personnel available to callers.*

People's Medical Society
462 Walnut Street, Lower Level
Allentown, PA 18102
800-624-8773
215-770-1670
8:30 a.m. to 5:00 p.m. (eastern time) Monday-Friday
Answering machine at all other times
> *Provides information on how to become a better informed medical consumer. Also publishes consumer-oriented medical information on topics ranging from pediatrics to Medicare. Free membership information and publication list available upon request.*

Total Health Foundation
P. O. Box 5
Yakima, WA 98907
800-348-0120
24 hours a day
> *Provides information on a variety of medical topics.*

HEARING IMPAIRMENTS

American Speech-Language-Hearing Association Helpline
10801 Rockville Pike
Rockville, MD 20852
800-638-8255 Voice- and hearing-impaired
800-897-8682 Alaska, Hawaii, and Maryland
301-897-8682
8:30 a.m. to 4:30 p.m. (eastern time) Monday-Friday
> *Provides general information on speech, language, and hearing problems and makes referrals to professionals. Free information packet available upon request.*

Better Hearing Institute
P. O. Box 1840
Washington, DC 20013
800-424-8576 Virginia
703-642-0580
9:00 a.m. to 5:00 p.m. (eastern time) Monday-Friday
> *Provides information on deafness and other types of hearing problems.*

Captioned Films for the Deaf
5000 Park Street North
St. Petersburg, FL 33709
800-237-6213
813-545-8781
> *Provides information on films that are available with captioning for the hearing impaired.*

Deafness Research Foundation
9 East 38th Street, 7th Floor
New York, NY 10016-0003
800-535-3323 Voice- and hearing-impaired
212-684-6556 New York City
9:00 a.m. to 5:00 p.m. (eastern time) Monday-Friday
> *Provides information on hearing problems and makes referrals to local physicians. Also provides information on how to select a hearing aid and detect hearing problems in children. Free materials available upon request.*

Delta Society
P. O. Box 1080
Renton, WA 98057-1080
800-869-6898
206-226-7357
> *Provides information on how to obtain hearing dogs for the deaf.*

Hear Now
4001 South Magnolia Way, Suite 100
Denver, CO 80237
800-648-4327 Voice- and hearing-impaired
303-758-4919 Colorado
8:30 a.m. to 4:00 p.m. (mountain time) Monday-Friday
Answering machine at all other times
> *Provides information on hearing aids and ear implants. Also sponsors a national hearing-aid bank and makes referrals to local organizations and agencies.*

Hearing Aid Hotline
20361 Middlebelt Road
Livonia, MI 48152
800-521-5247
313-478-2610
> *Provides information on hearing loss and hearing aids. Also makes referrals to hearing-aid specialists.*

Hearing Information Center
P. O. Box 1880
Media, PA 19063
800-622-3277
> *Provides hearing screening over the phone and also answers general questions about hearing.*

National Captioning Institute
5203 Leesburg Pike
Falls Church, VA 22041
800-533-9673
703-998-2443
> *Provides captioning services for television programs and films.*

Sensor Hearing Aids
300 South Chester Road
Swarthmore, PA 19081
800-622-3277
215-544-2700
9:00 a.m. to 5:00 p.m. (eastern time) Monday-Friday
Provides free information on hearing loss and hearing aids.
Also makes referrals to audiologists in caller's area.

TRIPOD Grapevine
2901 N. Keystone Street
Burbank, CA 91504
800-352-8888 Voice- and hearing-impaired
800 287-4763 Voice- and hearing-impaired (California)
9:00 a.m. to 5:00 p.m. (Pacific time) Monday-Friday
Provides information and services to parents who are raising a
hearing-impaired child.

HEART DISEASE

American Heart Association
7272 Greenville Avenue
Dallas, TX 75231
800-242-8721
Provides information on coronary conditions and makes referrals to
local support groups.

HOSPICE

Children's Hospice International
900 North Washington Street, Suite 700
Alexandria, VA 22314
800-242-4453
703-684-0330 Virginia
8:30 a.m. to 5:30 p.m. (eastern time) Monday-Friday
Answering machine at all other times
Provides information on hospice programs especially designed for
children with life-threatening conditions or who are terminally ill.

Hospice Education Institute
5 Essex Square
P. O. Box 713
Essex, CT 06246
800-544-2213
203-767-1620 Alaska and Connecticut
9:00 a.m. to 4:30 p.m. (eastern time) Monday-Friday
> *Provides information and counseling on death and dying and the role*
> *of the hospice. Also makes referrals to local agencies and publishes a*
> *directory of hospices.*

National Hospice Organization
1901 North Moore Street, Suite 901
Arlington, VA 22209
800-658-8898
8:30 a.m. to 5:30 p.m. (eastern time) Monday-Friday
> *Provides information on hospice programs available in the caller's area.*

HOSPITAL CARE

Hill-Burton Hospital Program
Division of Facilities Compliance
Parklawn Building, Room 11-25
5600 Fishers Lane
Rockville, MD 20857
800-638-0742
800-492-0359 Maryland
9:30 a.m. to 5:30 p.m. (eastern time) Monday-Friday
Answering machine at all other times
> *Provides information on hospitals that are participating in the*
> *Hill-Burton Free Care Program in the caller's area. Free information*
> *packet available upon request.*

HUNTINGTON'S DISEASE

Huntington's Disease Society of America
140 West 22nd Street, 6th Floor
New York, NY 10011-2420
800-345-4372
212-242-1968 New York
9:00 a.m. to 5:00 p.m. (eastern time) Monday-Friday
> *Provides information and referrals to individuals with Huntington's*
> *disease and their families. Also offers crisis intervention and makes*
> *referrals to support groups. Free information available upon request.*

INCONTINENCE

Simon Foundation for Continence
P. O. Box 815
Wilmette, IL 60091
800-237-4666
708-864-3913 Illinois
9:00 a.m. to 6:00 p.m. (central time) 7 days a week
Provides information on incontinence. Also makes referrals to specialists in the field and support groups in the caller's area.

INSURANCE

Alternative Health Insurance Services
P. O. Box 9178
Calabasas, CA 91372-9178
800-331-2713
818-509-5742 Los Angeles
Provides information on insurance plans that cover alternative health care practitioners.

Communicating for Seniors
P. O. Box 677
Fergus Falls, MN 56538
800-432-3276
8:00 a.m. to 4:30 p.m. (central time) Monday-Friday
Provides information on insurance matters to the elderly, especially in the area of Medicare supplemental insurance. Free information available upon request.

Coop-America
2100 M Street, N.W., Suite 403
Washington, DC 20037
800-424-2667
202-872-5200 District of Columbia
Provides information on worker-owned and cooperatively structured health insurance plans that provide coverage for conventional as well as alternative practitioners.

National Insurance Consumer Helpline
American Council of Life Insurance
Health Insurance Association of America
Insurance Information Institute
1001 Pennsylvania Avenue, N.W.
Washington, DC 20004
800-942-4242

> *Provides general information on how to choose an agent or broker and an insurance company. Also provides information on the following types of insurance: health, long-term-care, disability, Medicare supplemental, and major medical. Does not provide information on specific policies or companies.*

KIDNEY DISEASES

American Association of Kidney Patients
111 South Parker Street, Suite 405
Tampa, FL 33606
800-749-2257
813-251-0725 Tampa area
9:00 a.m. to 5:00 p.m. (eastern time) Monday-Friday

> *Provides information to kidney patients and their families on coping with kidney disease.*

American Kidney Fund
6110 Executive Boulevard, Suite 1010
Rockville, MD 20852
800-638-8299
800-492-8361 Maryland
8:00 a.m. to 5:00 p.m. (eastern time) Monday-Friday

> *Provides information on kidney diseases and organ donor programs. Also offers financial assistance to kidney patients. Public education materials available upon request.*

National Kidney Foundation
30 East 33rd Street
New York, NY 10016
800-622-9010
8:30 a.m. to 5:30 p.m. (eastern time) Monday-Friday

> *Provides information on research into kidney and urinary tract diseases, organ donations, and transplant programs. Also provides materials for public education programs.*

National Medical Care Patient Travel Service
Reservoir Place
1601 Trapelo Road
Waltham, MA 02154
800-634-6254

> *Provides information to dialysis patients on how to arrange for dialysis at a National Medical Center dialysis facility while on vacation.*

LIVER DISEASES

American Liver Foundation
1425 Pompton Avenue
Cedar Grove, NJ 07009
800-223-0179
201-857-2626 New Jersey
8:30 a.m. to 4:30 p.m. (eastern time) Monday-Friday
Provides information and assistance to children and adults with liver diseases. Also makes referrals to specialists and support groups.

LUNG DISEASES

Cystic Fibrosis Foundation
6931 Arlington Road
Bethesda, MD 20814
800-344-4823
301-951-4422
8:30 a.m. to 5:30 p.m. (eastern time) Monday-Friday
Provides information on cystic fibrosis and makes referrals to hospital treatment centers and local support groups. Free information available upon request.

LUPUS

Lupus Foundation of America
4 Research Place, Suite 180
Rockville, MD 20850-3226
800-558-0121
301-670-9292 Maryland
24 hours a day
Provides free information concerning books written by doctors and patients who have lupus and refers callers to local chapters of the Lupus Foundation.

Terri Gotthelf Lupus Research Institute
3 Duke Place
South Norwalk, CT 06854
800-825-8787
203-852-0120
9:00 a.m. to 7:30 p.m. (eastern time) Monday-Friday
Provides information on medical centers that conduct research into the cause and treatment of lupus. Also provides general information on lupus to patients and their families. Free information available upon request.

MEDIC ALERT

Medic Alert Foundation International
2323 North Colorado Avenue
Turlock, CA 95380
800-432-5378
800-468-1020 California
209-668-3333 Alaska and Hawaii
24 hours a day

> *Provides information on how to register with Medic Alert and obtain an emergency identification bracelet. Also maintains a record of the patient's medical record that can be retrieved in an emergency. Free registration form and catalog available upon request.*

MEDICARE/MEDICAID

Inspector General's Hotline
U.S. Department of Health and Human Services
P. O. Box 17303
Baltimore, MD 21203-7303
800-368-5779
800-638-3986 Maryland

> *Handles complaints from recipients relating to overcharges and possible fraud and waste of funds in the Medicare and Medicaid programs.*

Medicare Information Hotline
U.S. Department of Health and Human Services
Health Care Financing Administration
Washington, DC 20201
800-888-1770 Recorded message
800-888-1998 To request written material or ask questions
8:00 a.m. to midnight, 7 days a week.

> *Provides general information on the Medicare program and responds to specific questions concerning Medicare coverage.*

Medicare Medigap Insurance Fraud Line
U.S. Department of Health and Human Services
Health Care Financing Administration
Washington, DC 20201
800-638-6833

> *Provides information on the new Medicare supplemental, or medigap, policies and also receives complaints from beneficiaries concerning instances of medigap fraud and abuse.*

MEN'S HEALTH

Impotence Foundation
800-221-5517
9:00 a.m. to 5:00 p.m. (Pacific time) Monday-Friday
Provides information on the treatment of impotence.

Impotence Information Center
P. O. Box 9
Minneapolis, MN 55440
800-843-4315
8:00 a.m. to 5:30 p.m. (central time) Monday-Friday
Answering machine at all other times
Provides free information on the causes and treatments of impotence,
but does not provide on-line counseling. Also provides the names and
addresses of urologists in the caller's area.

Star Center
27211 Lahser Road, Suite 208
Southfield, MI 48034
800-835-7667
313-357-1314 Michigan
24 hours a day
Provides general information on impotency and makes referrals to
practitioners in the caller's area.

Us Too (Prostate Cancer)
American Foundation for Urologic Disease, Inc.
300 West Pratt Street, Suite 401
Baltimore, MD 21201
800-828-7866
Provides information on the latest developments in the diagnosis
and treatment of prostate cancer. Also makes referrals to local chapters
of Us Too.

MENTAL HEALTH

American Board of Professional Psychology
2100 East Broadway, Suite 313
Columbia, MO 65201-6082
800-255-7792
Provides information on psychologists who have met the standards
required for certification.

American Mental Health Counselors Association
5999 Stevenson Avenue
Alexandria, VA 22304
800-326-2642
703-823-9800
8:30 a.m. to 4:30 p.m. (eastern time) Monday-Friday
*Provides information on professionals in the counseling field and
makes local referrals.*

American Mental Health Fund
1021 Price Street
Alexandria, VA 22314
800-433-5959
703-684-2201 Virginia
24 hours a day
*Provides general information on mental illness. Callers may request
packets of information that include the location and telephone numbers
for local chapters.*

American Schizophrenic Association
900 North Federal Highway, Suite 330
Boca Raton, FL 33432
800-847-3802
24 hours a day
*Provides general information and educational materials about mental
illnesses and learning disabilities. Also makes referrals to physicians.
Free literature available upon request.*

Camelback Helpline
7575 East Earl Drive
Scottsdale, AZ 85251
800-253-1334
24 hours a day
*Provides information on such subjects as mental health, eating
disorders, and substance dependency. Makes referrals to treatment
centers nationwide. Free information available upon request.*

National Alliance for the Mentally Ill
2101 Wilson Boulevard, Suite 302
Arlington, VA 22201
800-950-6264
9:00 a.m. to 5:00 p.m. (eastern time) Monday-Friday
Answering machine at all other times
*Provides information on local chapters, advocacy, and support groups
for the mentally ill. Free literature available upon request.*

National Foundation for Depressive Illness
P. O. Box 2257
New York, NY 10116
800-248-4344
24 hours a day
*Provides general information on depression and directs the caller to
other organizations that can provide additional information on specific
conditions and physician referrals.*

National Mental Health Association
1021 Prince Street
Alexandria, VA 22314-2971
800-969-6642
703-684-7722 Virginia
9:00 a.m. to 6:00 p.m. (eastern time) Monday-Friday
*Provides information on mental health and mental illnesses. Also
makes referrals to local support groups, mental health centers, self-help
clearinghouses, and other organizations. Free packet of information
available upon request.*

MENTAL RETARDATION

American Association on Mental Retardation
1719 Kalorma Road, N.W.
Washington, DC 20009
800-424-3688
202-387-1968 District of Columbia
9:00 a.m. to 5:00 p.m. (eastern time) Monday-Friday
*Provides general information on mental retardation and makes
referrals to practitioners. Free information packet on the association's
services and publications available upon request.*

MULTIPLE SCLEROSIS
(MS)

National Multiple Sclerosis Society
733 Third Avenue
New York, NY 10017-3288
800-624-8236
212-986-3240 New York
24 hours a day
*Provides general information on multiple sclerosis and makes referrals
to local groups. Free information packet lists MS centers, board
certified neurologists, and updates on the latest research into the
causes and treatments of MS.*

MYASTHENIA GRAVIS
(MG)

Myasthenia Gravis Foundation
53 West Jackson Boulevard, Suite 660
Chicago, IL 60604
800-541-5454
8:00 a.m. to 5:00 p.m. (central time) Monday-Friday
Provides information on the diagnosis and treatment of MG and also makes referrals to local support groups.

NEUROFIBROMATOSIS

National Neurofibromatosis Foundation
141 Fifth Avenue, Suite 7-S
New York, NY 10010
800-323-7938
212-460-8980 New York
9:00 a.m. to 5:00 p.m. (eastern time) Monday-Friday
Provides information and assistance to neurofibromatosis patients and their families. Free information packet available upon request.

NUTRITION INFORMATION

Akpharma Foods, Inc.
P. O. Box 111
Pleasantville, NJ 08232-0111
800-257-8650
9:00 a.m. to 5:00 p.m. (eastern time) Monday-Friday
Provides information on a product that helps people digest beans and vegetable fiber. Free information and sample of the product available upon request.

American Dietetic Association
Consumer Nutrition Hotline
216 West Jackson Boulevard, Suite 800
Chicago, IL 60606
800-366-1655
10:00 a.m. to 5:00 p.m. (central time) Monday-Friday
Recorded messages 24 hours a day
Provides general information on nutrition, including cholesterol, weight control, and healthy snacks. Also makes referrals to nutritional counselors in the caller's area. Provides special service for teenagers.

American Institute for Cancer Research
AICR Nutrition Hotline
1759 R Street, N.W.
Washington, DC 20009
800-843-8114
202-328-7744 District of Columbia
9:00 a.m. to 9:00 p.m. (eastern time) Monday-Thursday
9:00 a.m. to 5:00 p.m. (eastern time) Friday
Answering machine at all other times
*Provides information on the relationship between diet and nutrition
and cancer. Callers may ask specific questions about cancer and diet.*

Beech-Nut Nutrition, Inc.
Checkerboard Square
Consumer Affairs, 1-B
St. Louis, MO 63164
800-523-6633
800-492-2384 Pennsylvania
9:00 a.m. to 8:00 p.m. (eastern time) Monday-Friday
*Provides information on nutritional content of baby food and answers
food-related questions.*

Gerber Hotline
Consumer Relations Gerber Products
445 State Street
Fremont, MI 49413
800-443-7237
Provides information on infant nutrition and specific baby-care topics.

HCF Foundation
High Carbohydrate Fiber
University of Kentucky
800 Rose Street
Lexington, KY 40536
800-727-4423
*Provides information on the role of fiber in the diet as it relates to
cholesterol, diabetes, and blood sugar levels. Callers may leave specific
questions on voice-mail system.*

International Olive Oil Council
P. O. Box 2506
Stuart, FL 34995-2506
800-232-6548
9:00 a.m. to 5:00 p.m. (eastern time) Monday-Friday
*Provides information on the nutritional and fat content of olive oil.
Free information available upon request.*

Lactaid, Inc.
McNeil Consumer Affairs
P. O. Box 85
Camp Hill Road
Ft. Washington, PA 19034
800-522-8243
9:00 a.m. to 5:00 p.m. (eastern time) Monday-Friday
> *Provides information on Lactaid and lactose intolerance.*
> *Free information and samples available upon request.*

Meat and Poultry Hotline
U.S. Department of Agriculture
Room 1165 S, FSIS
Washington, DC 20250
800-535-4555
202-720-3333 District of Columbia
10:00 a.m. to 4:00 p.m. (eastern time) Monday-Friday
> *Provides information on the proper handling and storage of meat*
> *and poultry products. Free information available upon request.*

Molly McButter Information Hotline
800-622-3274
9:00 a.m. to 5:00 p.m. (eastern time) Monday-Friday
> *Provides information on the fat and calorie content of foods.*
> *Callers may ask questions of registered dietitians.*

Mrs. Dash Sodium Information Hotline
800-622-3274
9:00 a.m. to 5:00 p.m. (eastern time) Monday-Friday
> *Provides low-sodium recipes and information on the sodium content of*
> *foods for people on sodium-restricted diets. Free information available*
> *upon request.*

Seafood Hotline
U.S. Department of Health and Human Services
Food and Drug Administration
Rockville, MD 20857
800-FDA-4010
202-205-4314 District of Columbia
10:00 a.m. to 2:00 p.m. (eastern time) Monday-Friday
Answering machine at all other times
> *Provides information on how to buy and use seafood products. Callers*
> *may speak to food specialists during the hours shown above. At all*
> *other times callers may access prerecorded information on the proper*
> *handling and storage of seafood. List of FDA seafood publications is*
> *also available from the hotline.*

ORGAN DONOR PROGRAMS

The Living Bank
P. O. Box 6725
Houston, TX 77265
800-528-2971
713-528-2971 Texas
24 hours a day
> *Operates a registry and referral program for people wishing to donate their vital organs or bodies to research.*

National Marrow Donor Program
3433 Broadway Street N.E., Suite 400
Minneapolis, MN 55413
800-654-1247
8:00 a.m. to 5:00 p.m. (central time) Monday-Friday
Answering machine at all other times
> *Provides information on how to become a bone marrow donor. Also maintains a national registry of volunteers. Free information available upon request.*

Organ Donor Hotline
United Network for Organ Sharing
1100 Boulders Parkway, Suite 500
P. O. Box 13770
Richmond, VA 23225-8770
800-243-6667
804-330-8500
9:00 a.m. to 5:00 p.m. (eastern time) Monday-Friday
> *Provides information on organ donor programs and transplants. Also provides organ donor cards upon request.*

ORPHAN DRUGS AND RARE DISEASES

Friends of Karen
P. O. Box 217
Croton Falls, NY 10519
800-637-2774
9:00 a.m. to 5:00 p.m. (eastern time) Monday-Friday
> *Provides information on financial support that may be available to families with children who have life-threatening or rare diseases. Also provides information on support groups to aid the families. Free information available upon request.*

National Information Center for Orphan Drugs and Rare Diseases
P. O. Box 1133
Washington, DC 20013
800-336-4797
202-429-9091 District of Columbia
9:00 a.m. to 5:00 p.m. (eastern time) Monday-Friday
Provides information on how to locate a source for orphan drugs. (Orphan drugs, for which there is only a small market, are used to treat rare illnesses.)

National Information Clearinghouse for Infants With Disabilities and Life-Threatening Conditions
University of South Carolina
Benson Building, 1st Floor
Columbia, SC 29208
800-922-9234 Voice- and hearing-impaired
800-922-1107 Voice- and hearing-impaired (South Carolina)
9:00 a.m.. to 5:00 p.m. (eastern time) Monday-Friday
Answering machine at all other times
Provides information to families with children who have rare or life-threatening conditions. Also makes referrals to professional and community services in the caller's area. Offers special services to Vietnam veterans and their families.

National Organization for Rare Disorders
P. O. Box 8923
New Fairfield, CT 06812-1783
800-447-6673
9:00 a.m. to 5:00 p.m. (eastern time) Monday-Friday
Answering machine at all other times
Provides information on how individuals may apply for the drug cost-sharing program that the pharmaceutical industry sponsors to help consumers pay the cost of medications. Free information available upon request.

OSTEOPOROSIS

National Osteoporosis Foundation
2100 M Street, N.W., Suite 602-B
Washington, DC 20037
800-223-9994
Provides information on osteoporosis, including a publication answering basic questions about the condition. Free information packet available upon request.

PARALYSIS AND SPINAL CORD INJURY

APA Spinal Cord Injury Hotline
2201 Argonne Drive
Baltimore, MD 21218
800-526-3456
8:30 a.m. to 5:30 p.m. (eastern time) Monday-Friday
Answering machine at all other times
> *Provides information on spinal cord injuries and referrals to local*
> *organizations, agencies, and treatment centers.*

American Paralysis Association
Montebello Hospital
500 Morris Avenue
Springfield, NJ 07081
800-225-0292
201-379-2690 New Jersey
8:30 a.m. to 5:00 p.m (eastern time) Monday-Friday
> *Provides information on research into treatment of spinal cord injuries*
> *and prospects for recovery. Free information available upon request.*

National Spinal Cord Injury Association
600 West Cummings Park, Suite 2000
Woburn, MA 01801
800-962-9629
617-935-2722 Massachusetts
9:00 a.m. to 5:00 p.m. (eastern time) Monday-Friday
> *Provides information for patients and their families on services*
> *available from organizations, agencies, and local support groups.*
> *Free information packet available upon request.*

PARENTING

A Way Out
7 Innis Avenue
New Paltz, NY 12561
800-292-9688
914-255-1907
> *Provides 24-hour-a-day assistance to parents who are considering*
> *abducting their children or who already have taken their children.*

Father Advocacy Information Referral
140-B Sandune Drive
Pittsburgh, PA 15239
800-722-3247
> *Provides assistance with visitation rights and custody for*
> *divorced fathers.*

Foster Parents Plan
155 Plan Way
Warwick, RI 02886
800-556-7918
Provides information on becoming a foster parent.

National Association for Parents of the Visually Impaired
P. O. Box 317
Watertown, MA 02272-0317
800-562-6265
608-362-4945 Wisconsin
9:00 a.m to 5:00 p.m. (central time) Monday-Friday
Provides general information and counseling to families with visually impaired children.

Parents Anonymous/Abusive Parents
520 South Lafayette Park Place, Suite 316
Los Angeles, CA 90057
800-421-0353
800-352-0386 California
Provides assistance and counseling to parents who have been involved in child abuse or abusive situations.

Parents Without Partners
8807 Colesville Road
Silver Spring, MD 20910
800-637-7974
301-588-9354 Maryland
Provides information on area support groups for single parents.

Technical Assistance to Parent Programs Network
Federation for Children With Special Needs
95 Berkeley Street, Suite 104
Boston, MA 02116
800-331-0688 Massachusetts
9:00 a.m. to 5:00 p.m. (eastern time) Monday-Friday
Provides information to parents with children who have special needs because of developmental disabilities. Also provides information on special education laws, and provides training and workshops for parents of children with special needs. Makes referrals to a national network of support groups.

Toughlove, Inc.
P. O. Box 1069
Doylestown, PA 18901
800-333-1069
215-348-7090 Pennsylvania
Provides information on psychological treatment programs for children with behavioral problems.

PARKINSON'S DISEASE

American Parkinson's Disease Association
60 Bay Street, Suite 401
Staten Island, NY 18901
800-223-2732 New York
9:00 a.m. to 5:00 p.m. (eastern time) Monday-Friday
Answering machine at all other times
> *Provides brochures and sends information on medicines used to treat Parkinson's. Also offers counseling services and makes referrals to treatment centers.*

National Parkinson's Foundation
1501 N.W. 9th Avenue
Miami, FL 33136
800-327-4545
800-433-7022 Florida
305-547-6666 Miami area
8:00 a.m. to 5:00 p.m. (eastern time) Monday-Friday
> *Provides information on Parkinson's disease and makes referrals to physicians.*

Parkinson's Disease Foundation
William Black Medical Research Building
650 West 168th Street
New York, NY 10032
800-457-6676
9:00 a.m. to 5:00 p.m. (eastern time) Monday-Friday
> *Provides information on patient care and rehabilitation, including lists of self-help groups and of clinics where treatment is available. Publishes newsletter four times a year. Clinical specialists available to answer questions.*

Parkinson's Education Program
3900 Birch Street, Suite 105
Newport Beach, CA 92660
800-344-7872
714-640-0218 California
24 hours a day
> *Provides written materials, including newsletters and other publications and definitions of key terms. Also makes referrals to support groups. Caller may leave name and address to receive materials.*

PESTICIDES

National Pesticides Information Clearinghouse
National Pesticides Telecommunications Network
Texas Tech University
Health Science Center/Department of Preventative Medicine
Lubbock, TX 79430
800-858-7378
800-292-7664 Texas
24 hours a day
> *Provides information to the public and the medical profession on the
> hazards of pesticides.*

PHYSICIAN CREDENTIALING

ABMS Certification Line
American Board of Medical Specialties
180 Allen Road, Suite 302
Atlanta, GA 30328
800-776-2378
9:00 a.m. to 6:00 p.m. (eastern time) Monday-Friday
> *Provides information on the certification status of physicians,
> including their specialty and year certified. Caller should have
> physician's name and location ready before calling.*

POISON CONTROL CENTERS
(Only available in state shown)

See also: **PESTICIDES** and **TOXIC SUBSTANCES**

Note: *If a number is not listed for your state, contact the hospitals
serving your area.*

ALABAMA

Alabama Poison Center
809 University Boulevard East
Tuscaloosa, AL 35401
800-462-0800

Regional Poison Center
Children's Hospital of Alabama
1600 Seventh Avenue South
Birmingham, AL 35233
800-292-6678

ALASKA

Anchorage Poison Center
Providence Hospital
3200 Providence Drive
P. O. Box 196604
Anchorage, AK 99519-6604
800-478-3193

ARIZONA

Arizona Poison and Drug Information Center
University of Arizona
Arizona Health Science Center, Room 320-K
1501 North Campbell Avenue
Tucson, AZ 85724
800-362-0101
602-626-6016 Tucson

ARKANSAS

Arkansas Poison and Drug Information Center
University of Arkansas for Medical Sciences
College of Pharmacy, Slot 522
4301 West Markham Street
Little Rock, AR 72205
800-482-8948

CALIFORNIA

Fresno Regional Poison Control Center
Fresno Community Hospital and Medical Center
Fresno and R Streets
P. O. Box 1232
Fresno, CA 93715
800-346-5922 Fresno, Kern, Kings, Madera, Mariposa, Merced,
    and Tulare counties

Los Angeles County
Regional Poison Control Center
1925 Wilshire Boulevard
Los Angeles, CA 90057
800-777-6476 Los Angeles, Ventura, and Santa Barbara counties

San Diego Regional Poison Center
University of California
San Diego Medical Center
225 Dickinson Street, MC 8925
San Diego, CA 92103-8925
800-876-4766 Imperiale and San Diego counties

San Francisco Bay Area
Regional Poison Control Center
San Francisco General Hospital
1001 Potrero Avenue, Room 1E86
San Francisco, CA 94110
800-523-2222 Accessible in area codes 415, 510, and 707

Santa Clara Valley Medical Center
Regional Poison Center
751 South Bascom Avenue
San Jose, CA 95128
800-662-9886 Monterey, San Benito, San Louis Obispo,
   Santa Clara, and Santa Cruz counties

University of California-Davis Medical Center
Regional Poison Control Center
2315 Stockton Boulevard, Room 1511
Sacramento, CA 95817
800-342-9293

University of California-Irvine
Regional Poison Center
101 The City Drive, Route 78
Orange, CA 92668
800-544-4404 Inyo, Mono, Orange, Riverside, and
   San Bernadino counties

COLORADO

Rocky Mountain Poison and Drug Center
645 Bannock Street
Denver, CO 80204-4507
800-332-3070 Colorado
303-629-1123 Denver
800-525-5042 Montana
800-446-6179 Las Vegas, NV

CONNECTICUT

Connecticut Poison Control Center
University of Connecticut
Health Center
Farmington, CT 06030
800-343-2722

FLORIDA

**Florida Poison Information Center at
Tampa General Hospital**
Davis Island
P. O. Box 1289
Tampa, FL 33601
800-282-3171

GEORGIA

**Georgia Regional Poison Control Center
Grady Memorial Hospital**
80 Butler Street S.E.
Box 26066
Atlanta, GA 30335-3801
800-282-5846

HAWAII

**Hawaii Poison Center
Kapiolani Memorial Center for Women and Children**
1319 Punahou Street
Honolulu, HI 96826
800-362-3585

IDAHO

**Idaho Emergency Medical and Poison Control Center
St. Alphonsus Regional Medical Center**
1055 North Curtis Road
Boise, ID 83706
800-632-8000

ILLINOIS

**Central and Southern Illinois
Regional Poison Resource Center
St. John's Hospital**
800 East Carpenter Street
Springfield, IL 62769
800-252-2022 Central and southern Illinois

**Chicago and Northeastern Illinois
Regional Poison Control Center
Rush-Presbyterian-St. Luke's Medical Center**
1753 West Congress Parkway
Chicago, IL 60612
800-942-5969 Accessible in area codes 312, 708, 815, and 309

INDIANA

Indiana Poison Control Center
Methodist Hospital of Indiana
1701 North Senate Boulevard
P. O. Box 1367
Indianapolis, IN 46206
800-382-9097 Northern Indiana, northern Ohio, central and
   southern Michigan

IOWA

Poison Control Center
University of Iowa Hospitals and Clinics
200 Hawkins Drive
Iowa City, IA 52242
800-272-6477 Iowa, Minnesota, and Nebraska

Variety Club Poison and Drug Information Center
Iowa Methodist Medical Center
1200 Pleasant Street
Des Moines, IA 50309
800-362-2327

KANSAS

Mid-America Poison Center
University of Kansas Medical Center
3900 Rainbow, Room B-400
Kansas City, KS 66160
800-332-6633

KENTUCKY

Kentucky Regional Poison Center
Kosair Children's Hospital
P. O. Box 35970
Louisville, KY 40232-5070
800-722-5725
502-589-8222 Metropolitan Louisville and southern Indiana

MAINE

Maine Poison Control Center
Maine Medical Center
22 Bramhall Street
Portland, ME 04102
800-442-6305

MARYLAND

Maryland Poison Center
University of Maryland School of Pharmacy
20 North Pine Street
Baltimore, MD 21201
800-492-2414

MASSACHUSETTS

Massachusetts Poison Control System
300 Longwood Avenue
Boston, MA 02115
800-682-9211

MICHIGAN

Blodgett Regional Poison Center
Blodgett Memorial Medical Center
1840 Wealthy Street S.E.
Grand Rapids, MI 49506
800-632-2727
800-356-3232 Hearing impaired

Bronson Poison Center
Bronson Methodist Hospital
252 East Lowell Street
Kalamazoo, MI 49007
800-442-4112 Also serves northern Ohio and northern Indiana

MINNESOTA

Minnesota Regional Poison Center
St. Paul-Ramsey Medical Center
640 Jackson Street
St. Paul, MN 55101
800-222-1222 Excluding Anoka, Carver, Henaepin, and
  Scott counties

MISSOURI

Cardinal Glennon Children's Hospital
Regional Poison Center
1465 South Grand Boulevard
St. Louis, MO 63104
800-366-8888 Also serves western Illinois, Missouri, and
  Topeka, KS

MONTANA

Rocky Mountain Poison and Drug Center
645 Bannock Street
Denver, CO 80204-4507
800-525-5042

NEBRASKA

The Poison Center
Children's Memorial Hospital
8301 Dodge Street
Omaha, NE 68114
800-955-9119 Nebraska and Wyoming

NEW HAMPSHIRE

New Hampshire Poison Information Center
Dartmouth/Hitchcock Medical Center
1 Medical Center Drive
Lebanon, NH 03756
800-562-8236

NEW JERSEY

New Jersey Poison Information and Education System
Newark Beth Israel Medical Center
201 Lyons Avenue
Newark, NJ 07112
800-962-1253

NEW MEXICO

New Mexico Poison and Drug Information Center
University of New Mexico, North Campus
Albuquerque, NM 87131
800-432-6866
505-843-2551 Albuquerque

NEW YORK

Central New York Poison Control Center
University Hospital at Syracuse
750 East Adams Street
Syracuse, NY 13210
800-252-5655 All counties except Onodaga county

Hudson Valley Regional Poison Center
Nyack Hospital
North Midland Avenue
Nyack, NY 10960
800-336-6997

Life Line/Finger Lakes
Regional Poison Control Center
University of Rochester Medical Center
601 Elmwood Avenue, Box 321
Rochester, NY 14642
800-333-0542 Chemung, Livingston, Monroe, Ontario, Schuyer,
  Seneca, Steuben, Wayne, and Yates counties

Western New York Regional Poison Control Center
Children's Hospital of Buffalo
219 Byrant Street
Buffalo, NY 14222
800-888-7655

NORTH CAROLINA

Duke University Poison Control Center
P. O. Box 3007 DUMC
Durham, NC 27710
800-672-1697

Triad Poison Center
Moses H. Cone Memorial Hospital
1200 North Elm Street
Greensboro, NC 27401-1020
800-722-2222 Alamance, Forsyth, Guilford, Randolph, and
  Rockingham counties

Western North Carolina Poison Center
Memorial Mission Hospital
509 Biltmore Avenue
Asheville, NC 28801
800-542-4225

NORTH DAKOTA

North Dakota Poison Information Center
St. Luke's Hospital
720 4th Street North
Fargo, ND 58122
800-732-2200

OHIO

Akron Regional Poison Control Center
Children's Hospital Medical Center of Akron
281 Locust Street
Akron, OH 44308
800-362-9922

Central Ohio Poison Control Center
Children's Hospital
700 Children's Drive
Columbus, OH 43205
800-682-7625

Mahoning Valley Poison Center
St. Elizabeth Hospital Medical Center
1044 Belmont Avenue
Youngstown, OH 44501
800-426-2348 Ashtabula, Columbiana, Mahoning, and Trumbull
counties. Also serves Lawrence and Mercer counties in
Pennsylvania.

Regional Poison Control System and Drug and Poison
Information Center
University of Cincinnati Medical Center
231 Bethesda Avenue, M.L. 144
Cincinnati, OH 45267-0144
800-872-5111

Western Ohio Poison and Drug Information Center
Children's Medical Center
1 Children's Plaza
Dayton, OH 45404
800-762-0727

OKLAHOMA

Oklahoma Poison Control Center
Children's Hospital of Oklahoma
940 N.E. 13th Street
Oklahoma City, OK 73104
800-522-4611
405-271-5454 Oklahoma City

OREGON

Oregon Poison Center
Oregon Health Services University
3181 S.W. Sam Jackson Park Road
Portland, OR 97201
800-452-7165

PENNSYLVANIA

Central Pennsylvania Poison Center
University Hospital
Milton S. Hershey Medical Center
University Drive
Hershey, PA 17033
800-521-6110

Northwest Regional Poison Center
St. Vincent's Hospital
232 West 25th Street
Erie, PA 16544
800-822-3232 Pennsylvania area codes 814 and 412.
    Also serves southwestern New York and northwestern Ohio.

Susquehanna Poison Center
Geisinger Medical Center
North Academy Road
Danville, PA 17822-2005
800-352-7001

SOUTH CAROLINA

Palmetto Poison Center
University of South Carolina
College of Pharmacy
Columbia, SC 29208
800-922-1116

SOUTH DAKOTA

McKennen Poison Control Center
800 East 21st Street
P. O. Box 5045
Sioux Falls, SD 57117-5045
800-952-0123
800-843-0505 Also serves Iowa, Minnesota, and Nebraska

St. Luke's Midland Poison Control Center
305 South State Street
Aberdeen, SD 57401
800-592-1889 Also serves Minnesota, North Dakota,
    and Wyoming

TENNESSEE

**Middle Tennessee Regional Poison/Clinical
    Toxicology Center**
501 Oxford House
1161 21st Avenue South
Nashville, TN 37232
800-288-9999 Accessible only in area code 615

TEXAS

**North Texas Poison Center
Parkland Hospital**
5201 Harry Hines Boulevard
P. O. Box 35926
Dallas, TX 75235
800-441-0040

UTAH

Intermountain Regional Poison Control Center
50 North Medical Drive
Salt Lake City, UT 84132
800-456-7707

VIRGINIA

University of Virginia Blue Ridge Poison Center
Blue Ridge Hospital, Box 67
Charlottesville, VA 22901
800-451-1428 Central, northern and western Virginia

**Virginia Poison Center
Virginia Commonwealth University**
Box 522, MCV Station
Richmond, VA 23298
800-552-6337

WASHINGTON

Central Washington Poison Center
Yakima Valley Memorial Hospital
2811 Tieton Drive
Yakima, WA 98902
800-572-9176

Mary Bridge Poison Center
Mary Bridge Children's Hospital
317 South K Street
Tacoma, WA 98405-0987
800-542-6319

Seattle Poison Center
Children's Hospital and Medical Center
4800 Sand Point Way N.E.
P. O. Box C-5371
Seattle, WA 98105-0371
800-732-6985

Spokane Poison Center
St. Luke's Hospital
South 711 Cowley
Spokane, WA 99202
800-572-5842

WEST VIRGINIA

West Virginia Poison Center
West Virginia University
School of Pharmacy
3110 MacCorkle Avenue S.E.
Charleston, WV 25304
800-642-3625

WYOMING

See: **Nebraska** and **South Dakota**

PREGNANCY SERVICES

Abortion Hotline
National Abortion Federation
1436 U Street, N.W.
Washington, DC 20009
800-772-9100
202-667-5881 District of Columbia
9:30 a.m. to 5:30 p.m. (eastern time) Monday-Friday
> *Provides information on services available at clinics in the caller's area.*
> *Also provides information on state laws applicable to abortion services.*

American Academy of Husband-Coached Childbirth
P. O. Box 5224
Sherman Oaks, CA 91413-5224
800-422-4784
818-788-6662 Sherman Oaks area
24 hours a day
> *Provides information on the Bradley method of childbirth and makes*
> *referrals to local instructors. Free information, including directory of*
> *instructors, available upon request.*

American Society for Psychoprophylaxis in Obstetrics/Lamaze
1101 Connecticut Avenue, N.W., Suite 700
Washington, DC 20036
800-368-4404
202-857-1128 District of Columbia
9:00 a.m. to 5:00 p.m. (eastern time) Monday-Friday
> *Provides information on the Lamaze technique and makes referrals to*
> *local centers.*

Be Healthy, Inc.: Positive Pregnancy and Parenting Fitness
51 Saltrock Road
Baltic, CT 06330
800-433-5523
203-822-8573 Connecticut
9:00 a.m. to 5:00 p.m. (eastern time) Monday-Friday
Answering machine at all other times
> *Provides information on pregnancy and parenting, including audio*
> *and visual aids. Free packet of information available upon request.*

Bethany Christian Services
901 Eastern Avenue N.E.
Grand Rapids, MI 49503
800-238-4269
9:00 a.m. to 5:00 p.m. (eastern time) Monday-Friday
> *Provides pregnancy testing, counseling services, and adoption services*
> *to pregnant women.*

Birthright
686 North Broad Street
Woodbury, NJ 08096
800-848-5683
609-848-1818 New Jersey
8:00 a.m. to 3:00 p.m. (eastern time) Monday-Friday
Provides confidential pregnancy counseling to girls who are homeless because of their pregnancy. Also provides maternity and baby clothes and support services, such as medical and financial referrals.

Edna Gladney Center Pregnancy Hotline
2300 Hemphill
Ft. Worth, TX 76110
800-452-3639
817-926-3304 Texas
9:00 a.m. to 5:00 p.m. (central time) Monday-Saturday
Provides information on all the options of pregnancy, especially adoption. Residential services are provided to women who are considering placing their babies for adoption.

International Childbirth Education Association
P. O. Box 20048
Minneapolis, MN 55420
800-624-4934
Provides information on pregnancy, childbirth, and other related infant-health needs. Also operates a book center. Free information and catalog available upon request.

La Leche League International
P. O. Box 1209
9616 Minneapolis Avenue
Franklin Park, IL 60131-8209
800-525-3243
9:00 a.m. to 3:00 p.m. (central time) Monday-Friday
Provides information on breast feeding.

Planned Parenthood Federation
810 Seventh Avenue
New York, NY 10019
800-829-7732
212-541-7800 New York
8:30 a.m. to 5:00 p.m. (eastern time) Monday-Friday
Provides information on family planning matters, including the use of contraceptives. Makes referrals to Planned Parenthood clinics in the caller's area.

PREMENSTRUAL SYNDROME

PMS Access
P. O. Box 9326
Madison, WI 53715
800-222-4767
608-257-8682 Wisconsin
9:00 a.m. to 5:00 p.m. (central time) Monday-Friday
> *Provides information on all aspects of PMS. Makes referrals to physicians and clinics in the caller's area. Free information packet available upon request.*

PRODUCT SAFETY

U.S. Consumer Product Safety Commission
5401 Westbard Avenue
Bethesda, MD 20207
800-638-CPSC
800-638-8270 Hearing impaired
800-492-8104 Hearing impaired (Maryland)
9:00 a.m. to 5:00 p.m. (eastern time) Monday-Friday
> *Provides information on how to report complaints of injuries caused by consumer products.*

RETINITIS PIGMENTOSA
(RP)

National Retinitis Pigmentosa Foundation
1401 Mt. Royal Avenue, 4th Floor
Baltimore, MD 21217
800-683-5555
410-225-9400 Maryland
8:30 a.m. to 5:00 p.m. (eastern time) Monday-Friday
Answering machine at all other times
> *Provides information on the latest developments in the treatment of RP and answers questions.*

Retinitis Pigmentosa International Fighting Blindness
P. O. Box 900
Woodland Hills, CA 91367
800-344-4877
> *Provides information on RP and reports on research into the diagnosis and treatment of this condition.*

REYE'S SYNDROME

National Reye's Syndrome Foundation
426 North Lewis
P. O. Box 829
Bryan, OH 43506
800-233-7393
800-231-7393 Ohio
24 hours a day
> *Provides information on symptoms of Reye's syndrome and on treatment and support networks.*

SENIOR CITIZENS SERVICES

Alcohol Rehabilitation for the Elderly
Hopedale Medical Complex
P. O. Box 267
Hopedale, IL 61747
800-354-7089
800-344-0824 Illinois
24 hours a day
> *Provides information and also makes referrals to treatment programs for people aged 50 and older.*

Life Extension Foundation
2835 Hollywood Boulevard
P. O. Box 229120
Hollywood, FL 33022
800-327-6110
> *Provides information on anti-aging research.*

National Council on the Aging, Inc.
409 Third Street, S.W.
Washington, DC 20024
800-424-9046
202-479-1200 District of Columbia
9:00 a.m. to 5:00 p.m. (eastern time) Monday-Friday
> *Provides general information on the subject of aging. Also serves as a clearinghouse for other organizations that provide programs to the elderly. Free information packet available upon request.*

National Eye Care Project Hotline
P. O. Box 429098
San Francisco, CA 94142
800-222-3937
8:00 a.m. to 4:00 p.m. (Pacific time) Monday-Friday
> *Provides information on a program designed for senior citizens aged 65 or older who are considered economically disadvantaged. Income and resources test for eligibility. Makes referrals to medical professionals in the caller's area.*

SEXUALLY TRANSMITTED DISEASES

STD National Hotline
American Social Health Association
P. O. Box 13827
Research Triangle Park, NC 27709
800-227-8922
919-361-8400 North Carolina
8:00 a.m. to 11:00 p.m. (eastern time) Monday-Friday
> *Provides free and confidential information on sexually transmitted diseases. Also provides referrals for diagnosis and treatment.*

SKIN DISORDERS

American Society for Dermatological Surgery
930 North Meacham Road
Schaumburg, IL 60173
800-441-2737
9:00 a.m. to 5:00 p.m. (central time) Monday-Friday
> *Provides information on surgical procedures related to skin damage from the sun, disease, or aging. List of specialists in the caller's area available upon request.*

United Scleroderma Foundation
P. O. Box 350
Watsonville, CA 95077
800-722-4673
8:00 a.m. to 5:00 p.m. (Pacific time) Monday-Friday
> *Provides information on scleroderma and other related skin diseases. Makes referrals to local support groups and treatment centers.*

SLEEP DISORDERS

American Narcolepsy Association
P. O. Box 26230
San Carlos, CA 94126
800-222-6085
24 hours a day
Provides information on narcolepsy and makes local referrals.

Better Sleep Council
P. O. Box 13
Washington, DC 20044
800-827-5337
Provides guidelines to better sleeping.

SOCIAL SECURITY

National Association of Social Security
  Claimants Representatives
6 Prospect Street
Midland Park, NJ 07432
800-431-2804
914-735-8812 New York (call collect)
Provides the names of attorneys who specialize in Social Security cases.

Social Security Administration
Social Security Hotline
U.S. Department of Health and Human Services
6401 Security Boulevard
Baltimore, MD 21235
800-234-5772
7:00 a.m. to 7:00 p.m. (eastern time) Monday-Friday
Answering machine at all other times
*Provides information on Social Security claims and general
information concerning eligibility for the program.*

SPASMODIC TORTICOLLIS

National Spasmodic Torticollis Association, Inc.
P. O. Box 476
Elm Grove, WI 53122-0476
800-487-8385
24 hours a day
*Provides referrals to physicians and support groups. Free information
packet available upon request.*

SPEECH IMPAIRMENTS

American Speech-Language-Hearing Association Helpline
1081 Rockville Pike
Rockville, MD 20852
800-638-8255
8:30 a.m. to 4:30 p.m. (eastern time) Monday-Friday
> *Provides information on speech, hearing, and language problems.*
> *Makes referrals to professionals in the field of speech therapy.*
> *Free information available upon request.*

AT&T Special Needs Center
2001 Route 46, 3rd Floor
Parsippany, NJ 07054
800-833-3232
> *Provides information on purchasing or renting special equipment*
> *and services for speech- and hearing-impaired individuals.*

Institute of Logopedics
2400 Jardine Drive
Wichita, KS 67219
800-835-1043 (Includes Canada)
8:00 a.m. to 5:00 p.m. (central time) Monday-Friday
> *Provides information on services offered by the institute's outpatient*
> *audiology department.*

National Center for Stuttering
200 East 33rd Street, Suite 17-C
New York, NY 10016
800-221-2483
9:00 a.m. to 5:00 p.m. (eastern time) Monday-Friday
> *Provides information on methods used to treat stuttering in children*
> *and adults. Free information available upon request.*

SPINA BIFIDA

Spina Bifida Association of America
4590 MacArthur Boulevard, N.W., Suite 250
Washington, DC 20007
800-621-3141
301-770-7222 Maryland
9:00 a.m to 5:00 p.m. (eastern time) Monday-Friday
Answering machine at all other times
> *Provides free information on the birth defect spina bifida.*
> *Also makes referrals to local chapters.*

SPORTS MEDICINE

International Institute of Sports Science and Medicine
Center for Hip and Knee Surgery
1199 Hadley Road
Mooresville, IN 46158
800-237-7678 Indiana
> *Provides information on surgical procedures to repair hip and*
> *knee injuries.*

STROKE

Courage Stroke Network
3915 Golden Valley Road
Golden Valley, MN 55422
800-553-6321
612-588-0811 Minnesota
8:00 a.m. to 4:00 p.m. (central time) Monday-Friday
> *Provides consultation, information, public education, and referrals*
> *to local support groups.*

National Stroke Association
300 East Hampden Avenue, Suite 240
Englewood, CO 80110-2654
800-787-6537
8:00 a.m. to 5:00 p.m. (central time) Monday-Friday
> *Provides information on support networks for stroke victims and their*
> *families. Also serves as a clearinghouse of information on stroke,*
> *including referrals to local support groups.*

SUBSTANCE ABUSE: DRUGS AND ALCOHOL

Al-Anon Family Groups Headquarters
P. O. Box 862, Midtown Station
New York, NY 10018
800-356-9996
800-245-4656 New York
800-443-4525 Canada
9:00 a.m. to 5:00 p.m. (eastern time) Monday-Friday
> *Provides information on 12-step recovery programs for alcoholics and*
> *their families. Free information available upon request.*

Alcohol and Drug Referral Helpline
Highland Ridge Hospital
4578 South Highland Drive
Salt Lake City, UT 84117
800-821-4357
24 hours a day
> *Provides information on alcohol and drug abuse and also makes referrals to local support programs.*

Alcohol Helpline
Adcare Hospital of Worcester
107 Lincoln Street
Worcester, MA 01605
800-252-6465
24 hours a day
> *Provides basic information on alcohol treatment programs and makes referrals to local treatment facilities.*

Alcoholism and Drug Addiction Treatment Center
Scripps-Memorial Hospital
9904 Genesee Avenue
LaJolla, CA 92037
800-382-4357 California
619-457-4123
> *Provides information on substance-abuse programs and makes referrals to treatment services for adults and adolescents.*

American Council on Alcoholism
5024 Campbell Boulevard, Suite H
Baltimore, MD 21236
800-527-5344
410-931-9393 Baltimore area
9:00 a.m. to 5:00 p.m. (eastern time) Monday-Friday
Answering machine at all other times
> *Provides information on alcoholism prevention programs for adults and children. Also provides counseling and referrals to treatment programs.*

ASAP Treatment Hotline
31129 Via Colinas, Suite 701
Westlake Village, CA 91362
800-367-2727
> *Provides telephone counseling to callers and information on alcohol- and drug-rehabilitation programs.*

BABES World, Inc.
Beginning Alcohol and Addiction Basic Education Studies
17330 Northland Park Court
Southfield, MI 48075
800-542-2237
> *Provides information on alcohol- and drug-prevention programs designed for children.*

Cocaine Anonymous
3740 Overland Avenue, Suite G
Los Angeles, CA 90034
800-347-8998
310-559-5833 Los Angeles area
Provides information on cocaine addiction and rehabilitation programs.

Cottage Program International
57 West South Temple Street, Suite 420
Salt Lake City, UT 84101
800-752-6100
24 hours a day
Provides information on substance-abuse programs aimed at the family. Also makes referrals to local organizations and support groups.

Drug Abuse Information and Treatment Referral Line
National Institute on Drug Abuse
11426 Rockville Pike, Suite 410
Rockville, MD 20852
800-662-4357
800-662-9832 Spanish
800-228-0427 Hearing impaired
9:00 a.m. to 3:00 a.m. (eastern time) Monday-Friday
Noon to 3:00 a.m. (eastern time) Saturday and Sunday
Provides counseling and referral services to callers. Also provides general information on substance abuse and addiction.

Drug Abuse Resistance Education (DARE)
P. O. Box 2090
Los Angeles, CA 90051-0090
800-223-3273
Provides information on programs that teach people how to avoid using drugs and other harmful substances.

Families Anonymous
P. O. Box 528
Van Nuys, CA 91408
800-736-9805
818-989-7841
Provides information for families with children who have substance-abuse or behavioral problems. Also provides counseling for family members and friends.

Family Talk About Drinking
Anheuser-Busch Company
Department of Consumer Awareness and Education
One Busch Place
St. Louis, MO 63118
800-359-8255

> *Provides information to families on how to discuss alcohol use with young children and teenagers. Callers may request information booklets by leaving name and address on voice-mail system.*

Hazelton Foundation
15251 Pleasant Valley Road
P. O. Box 11
Center City, MN 55102
800-328-9000
800-262-5010 Minnesota
7:00 a.m. to 6:00 p.m. (central time) Monday-Friday
Answering machine at all other times

> *Provides information on substance-abuse treatment and rehabilitation programs and on publications for sale. Operates rehabilitation center and also makes referrals to other organizations and resources. Free information available upon request.*

Johnson Institute
7205 Ohms Lane
Minneapolis, MN 55439-2159
800-231-5165
800-247-0484 Minnesota

> *Provides educational materials and information on community substance-abuse prevention programs.*

Mothers Against Drunk Drivers (MADD)
511 East John Carpenter Freeway, Suite 700
Irving, TX 75062
800-438-6233
24 hours a day

> *Provides information on programs designed to prevent drunk driving.*

National Clearinghouse for Alcohol and Drug Information
6000 Executive Boulevard, Suite 402
Rockville, MD 20852
800-729-6686

> *Provides information and referrals to callers with questions about alcohol- and drug-treatment programs.*

National Cocaine Hotline
P. O. Box 100
Summit, NJ 07901-0100
800-262-2463

> *Provides information and referrals to drug-treatment and rehabilitation programs. Also answers specific questions on drug abuse.*

National Council on Alcoholism and Drug Dependence, Inc. Hopeline
12 West 21st Street
New York, NY 10010
800-622-2255
212-206-6770 New York area
24 hours a day

Provides referrals to local organizations and support groups. Callers may obtain the location of the nearest affiliate office by entering their zip code on the voice-mail system. Free information available upon request.

National Federation of Parents for a Drug-Free Youth
8730 Georgia Avenue, Suite 200
Silver Spring, MD 20910
800-554-5437

Provides information on programs designed to help parents and children prevent drug abuse. Also makes referrals to support groups.

National Parents Resources Institute for Drug Education
50 Hurt Plaza, Suite 210
Atlanta, GA 30303
800-677-7433
404-577-4500 Atlanta area

Provides information on starting community drug education programs for young people.

New Life (Women for Sobriety)
P. O. Box 618
Quakertown, PA 18951
800-333-1606
215-536-8026

Provides help and assistance to women alcoholics.

Pride Institute
14400 Martin Drive
Eden Prairie, MN 55344
800-547-7433
24 hours a day

Provides information for persons addicted to alcohol or drugs. Also makes referrals to treatment centers.

Target Resource Center
P. O. Box 20626
Kansas City, MO 64195
800-366-6667
8:00 a.m. to 4:30 p.m. (central time) Monday-Friday

Provides information on substance-abuse-avoidance programs designed for pre-school and school-age children, kindergarten through high school. Free catalog available upon request.

SUDDEN INFANT DEATH SYNDROME (SIDS)

American Sudden Infant Death Syndrome Institute
275 Carpenter Drive
Atlanta, GA 30328
800-232-7437
800-847-7437 Georgia
8:00 a.m. to 5:00 p.m. (eastern time) Monday-Friday
Answering machine at all other times
> *Provides information on research into the cause of SIDS and also provides counseling and referral services.*

Sudden Infant Death Syndrome Alliance
10500 Little Patuxent Parkway, Suite 420
Columbia, MD 21044
800-221-7437
8:00 a.m. to 5:00 p.m. (eastern time) Monday-Friday
Answering machine at all other times
> *Provides information to parents of young infants and also offers counseling and support services to parents who have lost a child to SIDS.*

SURGERY SERVICES

American Academy of Cosmetic Surgery
401 North Michigan Avenue
Chicago, IL 60611
800-221-9808
8:00 a.m. to 5:00 p.m. (central time) Monday-Friday
> *Provides information on cosmetic surgery and also makes referrals to physician members of the academy in the caller's area.*

American Academy of Facial Plastic and Reconstructive Surgeons
1110 Vermont Avenue, N.W., Suite 220
Washington, DC 20005
800-332-3223
800-532-3223 Canada
202-842-4500 District of Columbia
24 hours a day
> *Provides general information on plastic surgery. Callers may request lists of surgeons in their areas.*

American Association of Oral and Maxillofacial Surgeons
9700 Bryn Mawr Avenue
Rosemont, IL 60018
800-467-5268
8:30 a.m. to 5:00 p.m. (central time) Monday-Friday
Answering machine at all other times
Provides information and referrals to oral surgeons.

American Plastic Surgery Information
6707 First Avenue South
St. Petersburg, FL 33707
800-522-2222 Florida
Provides information on plastic and reconstructive surgery and makes referrals in caller's area.

American Society of Plastic and Reconstructive Surgeons
444 East Algonquin Road
Arlington Heights, IL 60005
800-635-0635
8:30 a.m. to 4:30 p.m. (central time) Monday-Friday
Provides information on surgical procedures and makes referrals to specialists within specified geographical areas. Also verifies credentials of plastic surgeons.

Plastic and Aesthetic Surgery Center
217 East Chestnut Street
Louisville, KY 40202
800-327-3613
800-633-8923 Kentucky
24 hours a day
Provides information about various plastic surgery procedures, including cost estimates. Also makes local referrals.

TOURETTE SYNDROME

Tourette Syndrome Association
42-40 Bell Boulevard
Bayside, NY 11361
800-237-0717
8:30 a.m. to 4:30 p.m. (eastern time) Monday-Friday
Answering machine at all other times
Provides information on the syndrome to patients and their families. Also makes referrals to local chapters in the caller's area.

TOXIC SUBSTANCES

Asbestos Technical Information Service
P. O. Box 12194
Research Triangle Park, NC 27709
800-334-8571
9:00 a.m. to 5:00 p.m. (eastern time) Monday-Friday
Provides information about different types of asbestos and proper removal and disposal procedures. Also provides information on home tests for asbestos.

Chemical Manufacturers Association
2501 M Street, N.W.
Washington, DC 20037
800-262-8200
202-887-1315 District of Columbia
9:00 a.m. to 6:00 p.m. (eastern time) Monday-Friday
Answering machine at all other times
Provides general information on the safe handling of chemicals. Makes referrals to the manufacturers of specific chemical products who are responsible for providing more detailed information on the proper use and safety of the product. Each company provides a fact sheet on the specific effects of exposure to the chemical.

Emergency Planning and Community Right-to-Know Information Hotline
U.S. Environmental Protection Agency
401 M Street, N.W.
Washington, DC 20460
800-535-0202
202-479-2449 District of Columbia
Provides information on chemicals used in the community and the workplace.

Environmental Defense Fund Hotline
1616 P Street, N.W.
Washington, DC 20036
800-225-5333
202-387-3500 District of Columbia
Provides information to the public on the issue of environmental protection, including ways in which individuals can help keep the environment clean.

National Center for Toxicological Research
NCTR Drive
Highway 365 North
County Road 3
Jefferson, AR 72079-9502
800-638-3321
Provides information on the effects of toxic substances on the environment.

TUBEROUS SCLEROSIS

National Tuberous Sclerosis Association
8000 Corporate Drive, Suite 120
Landover, MD 20785
800-225-6872
301-459-9888 Maryland
9:00 a.m. to 5:00 p.m. (eastern time) Monday-Friday
Answering machine at all other times

> *Provides referrals to local representatives of the association and also provides information on parent-to-parent support networks. Free packet of materials available upon request.*

VIETNAM VETERANS

Agent Orange Veteran Payment Program
P. O. Box 110
Hartford, CT 06104
800-225-4712
800-922-9234 Birth defect information line
8:00 a.m. to 6:00 p.m. (eastern time) Monday-Friday

> *Provides counseling and assistance to Vietnam veterans who are involved in the class action lawsuit against the manufacturers of the defoliant Agent Orange. Also provides information and counseling to families with children who have disabilities that may be linked to Agent Orange.*

Vietnam Veterans Agent Orange Victims, Inc.
P. O. Box 2465
Darien, CT 06820-0465
800-521-0198
9:00 a.m. to 4:00 p.m. (eastern time) Monday-Friday

> *Provides medical and legal advice, information, and counseling to veterans who were exposed to the defoliant Agent Orange. Has established a children's fund to aid families whose children may be suffering from birth defects and developmental disabilities linked to Agent Orange.*

VISION IMPAIRMENTS

> *See also:* **RETINITIS PIGMENTOSA**

American Council of the Blind
1155 Vermont Avenue, N.W., Suite 720
Washington, DC 20005
800-424-8666
202-467-5081 District of Columbia
3:00 p.m. to 5:30 p.m. (eastern time) Monday-Friday
Provides information and referrals to clinics, organizations, and government agencies that provide services to the blind.

American Foundation for the Blind
15 West 16th Street
New York, NY 10011
800-232-5463
8:30 a.m. to 4:30 p.m. (eastern time) Monday-Friday
Provides answers to questions concerning vision loss and blindness. Free information available upon request.

AT&T National Special Needs Center
2001 Route 46, 3rd Floor
Parsippany, NJ 07054
800-833-3232
Provides information on equipment that can be adapted to meet the needs of the visually impaired.

Audio Reader
P. O. Box 847
Lawrence, KS 66044
800-772-8898 Kansas
Provides information on reading services available to the visually impaired.

Blind Children's Center
4120 Marathon Street
Los Angeles, CA 90029-0159
800-222-3566
800-222-3567 California
Provides information on blindness and makes referrals to local organizations and support groups.

Books on Tape
P. O. Box 7900
Newport Beach, CA 92658-7900
800-626-3333
Provides information on talking books that may be rented or purchased.

Guide Dog Foundation for the Blind
371 East Jericho Turnpike
Smithtown, NY 11787
800-548-4337
9:00 a.m. to 5:00 p.m. (eastern time) Monday-Friday
Provides information on guide dogs and refers callers to local organizations.

International Orthokeratology Society
1575 West Big Beaver Road
Troy, MI 48084
800-626-7846
8:00 a.m. to 5:00 p.m. (eastern time) Monday-Friday
10:00 a.m. to 2:00 p.m. (eastern time) Saturday
Answering machine at all other times
Provides information on the use of contact lenses to correct astigmatism and myopia. Makes referrals in caller's local area. Free brochure and other information available upon request.

Job Opportunities for the Blind
National Federation of the Blind
1800 Johnson Street
Baltimore, MD 21230
800-638-7518
8:00 a.m. to 5:00 p.m. (eastern time) Monday-Friday
Provides career counseling, job listings, and referrals to the visually impaired who are seeking employment.

Library of Congress
National Service for the Blind and Physically Handicapped
1291 Taylor Street, N.W.
Washington, DC 20542
800-424-8567
202-794-8650 District of Columbia
Provides information on libraries that offer talking books and books in braille.

National Society to Prevent Blindness
National Center for Sight
500 East Remington Road
Schaumburg, IL 60173
800-221-3004
9:00 a.m. to 4:00 p.m. (central time) Monday-Friday
Provides literature on specific vision problems and conditions. Also produces educational materials and offers professional education programs.

WOMEN'S HEALTH

American College of Obstetricians and Gynecologists
409 12th Street, S.W.
Washington, DC 20024
800-673-8444
202-638-5577 District of Columbia
> *Provides information and educational materials on health issues related to obstetrics and gynecology.*

Breast Implant Information Service
Food and Drug Administration
P. O. Box 1802
Rockville, MD 20704-1802
800-532-4440
800-688-6167 Hearing impaired
9:00 a.m. to 7:00 p.m. (eastern time) Monday-Friday
Answering machine at all other times
> *Provides information on the status of clinical studies being conducted on the safety of silicone gel-filled breast implants. Free packet of information available upon request.*

Johnson and Johnson, Inc.
Personal Products Consumer Response Center
New Brunswick, NJ 08901
800-526-3967
> *Provides information on a wide range of women's health concerns, including toxic shock syndrome.*

Women's Sports Foundation
342 Madison Avenue, Suite 728
New York, NY 10173
800-227-3988
9:00 a.m. to 5:00 p.m. (eastern time) Monday-Friday
> *Provides information on women and sports, physical fitness, and sports medicine.*

INDEX AND
SUBJECT CROSS-REFERENCE

C

Cancer 20
Captioned Films *See* Vision Impairments
Cerebral Palsy 22
Chemical Hazards *See* Toxic Substances and Pesticides
Child Abuse *See* Children's Services, Domestic Violence, and Parenting
Child Nutrition *See* Nutrition Information
Child Pornography *See* Children's Services
Child Sexual Abuse *See* Children's Services
Child Substance Abuse *See* Substance Abuse
Childbirth *See* Pregnancy Services
Childhood Cancer *See* Cancer
Children's Services 22
Cleft Palate 27
Cocaine Abuse *See* Substance Abuse
Colitis *See* Digestive Diseases
Communication Systems *See* Handicapped Services and Emergency Medical Communication Systems
Computer Systems *See* Handicapped Services
Cooley's Anemia *See* Anemia
Cornelia de Lange Syndrome 27
Cosmetic Surgery *See* Surgery Services
Craniofacial Deformities *See* Surgery Services
Crohn's Disease *See* Digestive Diseases
Cystic Fibrosis *See* Lung Diseases

D

Deaf Children *See* Hearing Impairments
Deafness *See* Hearing Impairments
Dental Care 27
Depression *See* Mental Health
Dermatology *See* Skin Disorders
Developmental Disabilities *See* Handicapped Services, Mental Retardation, and Parenting
Diabetes Mellitus 28
Dietary Supplements *See* Nutrition Information
Dieting *See* Eating Disorders
Digestive Diseases 28
Disabilities *See* Handicapped Services
Domestic Violence 29 *See* also Parenting
Down Syndrome 30

T

V

W

150
WAYS TO BE A
SAVVY MEDICAL
CONSUMER

**≡People's
Medical
Society.**

OTHER BOOKS FROM
THE PEOPLE'S MEDICAL SOCIETY

Take This Book to the Hospital With You

How to Evaluate and Select a Nursing Home

Medicine on Trial

Medicare Made Easy

Your Medical Rights

Getting the Most for Your Medical Dollar

Take This Book to the Gynecologist With You

Take This Book to the Obstetrician With You

Healthy Body Book: Test Yourself for Maximum Health

Blood Pressure: Questions You Have ... Answers You Need

Your Heart: Questions You Have ... Answers You Need

The Consumer's Guide to Medical Lingo

150 Ways to Be a Savvy Medical Consumer

100 Ways to Live to 100

Take This Book to the Pediatrician With You

150
WAYS TO BE A
SAVVY MEDICAL
CONSUMER

By Charles B. Inlander
President, People's Medical Society
and
The Staff of the
People's Medical Society

People's
Medical
Society.

Allentown, PA

ISBN 0-9627334-5-8

CONTENTS

It takes a savvy consumer to cut through the maze known as the American health care system. But with the right information, the right attitude, and a willingness to be just a little assertive, you can get quality health care at a cost far less than what many of your friends and neighbors pay.

Despite all its virtues, all its miracles, and all its victories, our health care system is fraught with physical and economic dangers. It is a system that even renowned medical experts have labeled "out of control."

There are 37 million Americans without health insurance. Another 30 million people are underinsured – they could not cover their medical bills if confronted with a major illness or a prolonged medical encounter. Corporations, which once provided liberal health care benefits to employees at little or no cost, now require employees to pay part of their insurance premiums, deductibles, and copayments. Some companies even have cut their benefits.

The numbers tell the story. In 1990 America spent 12.5 percent of the gross national product, or GNP, on health care. That's $660 billion, or more than twice what we spent on national defense. It also represented a 10.5 percent increase over the previous year. Overall inflation for the same period was 6.1 percent (and is falling).

But if those numbers don't hit home, try these. The average American household spends $6,750 each year for health care services. This includes out-of-pocket payments to doctors and hospitals, insurance premiums, medical equipment purchases, federal and state taxes used for health care, and the cost of health care benefits built into the goods and services you buy.

Under normal economic circumstances, health care costs should be going down. Demand is nowhere near the level of supply. Approximately 40 percent of the hospital beds in this country are empty. Every one of America's major cities has a doctor glut—many more doctors than we need in order to provide quality care to consumers. A coronary bypass procedure, which has increased in frequency by more than 100 percent in the last 10 years, went from an average of $20,000 per procedure in 1980 to $40,000 in 1990. Yet in the 1970s, when that particular operation was coming into vogue, medical gurus were promising a dramatic drop in cost as the operation became more commonplace. That's a pretty serious medical misdiagnosis.

Even the quality of American medicine is coming into question. Hospital infections are rampant. One out of 10 people who enter a hospital today can expect to acquire an infection they did not have when they were admitted. That is an almost 100 percent increase in the last decade. Twenty percent of all people who enter a hospital acquire a condition while in the hospital that they did not have before they came. Several studies have shown that up to 40 percent of the people admitted to hospitals are there as a result of something a doctor has done to them.

And while Americans get the most health care in the world, and pay the highest fees for it, overall the nation ranks relatively low, compared to other countries, in such categories as length of life and infant mortality.

As a result, consumers now are taking a more "buyer beware" attitude about medical services. We are questioning more, saying no to what appear to be useless or unnecessary services, seeking second opinions, using outpatient services, and entering wellness and rehabilitation programs.

The federal government, insurers, and businesses have implemented programs that require patients to get preapproval for treatments to ensure that the consumer is getting the right treatment for the condition presented. Medicare beneficiaries are staying fewer days in the hospital than before. Insurance companies are encouraging use of less costly outpatient services. Businesses are telling their employees to use fewer medical services and use them only when absolutely necessary.

Yet medical inflation continues to race ahead of the general inflation rate. What has happened is that instead of letting the normal laws of economics prevail, the benevolent and compassionate men and women who practice medicine, operate hospitals, manufacture medical equipment, and make drugs are raising their prices to make up for lost traffic. They have decided that they deserve a certain (and continually rising) level of income and profit, no matter how few customers they have.

But doctors and other medical and health care professionals usually deny they are business types. They talk about caring, healing, touching, and compassion. They tell us how hard and how long they work, the sacrifices they make, the terrible trials and tribulations of a life in the service of the sick and needy. But consumers have come to understand that beneath the white coat, behind the surgical mask, between the two tubes of the stethoscope resides a businessperson. And consumers are asking for the information and tools to deal with these professionals in a businesslike way.

That is why we wrote this book. Medicine is a business. While it is a business that deals with illness and the human condition, we must remember economics is always at play. Every time we use medical services, there is a cost attached. Unless we have insurance, we may not be "accepted" by a hospital or doctor. Doctors have signs in their offices asking people to pay at the time of visit. Hospitals post notices about minimum fees for use of the emergency room. No matter how helpful a medical service may be, the business element is always involved.

For the past several years, there has been a movement among business and government to contain the cost of medical care. The reality is that the cost-containment strategies employed by business and government have been successful in containing costs—but only for some businesses and the federal government. It has had very little effect on the average consumer, employee, or Medicare beneficiary. In fact, cost containment has not meant a reduction in fees, but rather a reduction in the amount of money spent by parties trying to contain their costs.

Twenty-seven years ago, when the Medicare program was launched, Americans over the age of 65 were spending 15 percent of their incomes for medical services. That predicament was the impetus for passage of the Medicare legislation. Citizens were outraged at these costs, and the Medicare program came into being. However, by 1990 something astounding had occurred. Medicare beneficiaries were now spending upwards of 20 percent of their incomes on medical care over and above what Medicare covered. In other words, the very economic conditions elderly people confronted in 1965 that brought about Medicare were even worse in 1991.

So much for the bad news. Now, what do we do as medical consumers? First, we arm ourselves with information—facts and figures that help us find the best care at the best price. Second, we formulate the questions that will get us the substantive answers we need from our health care providers.

And here's the good news. In the pages that follow, we have listed and explained 150 ways to be a savvy medical consumer. We have given you the facts and information that will help you find the best health care at the lowest price. Some of what you read, you may already know. Other ideas may never have dawned on you.

Every one of the 150 ways to find quality health care and lower your health care costs listed in this book works. They have worked for others just like you.

As president of the People's Medical Society, I am convinced that as individuals we can have quality health care and keep our personal expenditures down. As I travel around the country speaking to tens of thousands of people each year, they tell me what they have done to reduce costs for themselves. We have listed those methods in this book.

This book is your key for entering the world of quality health care and reasonable medical costs. We have tried to give you real actions you can take to make sure you receive the best medical care at the best price. (And believe me, I know they work. I have tried many myself.)

The staff of the People's Medical Society and I have reviewed all of these ideas. They are winners. And you too can be a winner over medical incompetence and medical inflation.

Read these ideas carefully. Use them at the next appropriate time. You will be surprised at just how easy it is to take charge of your own medical care. Do not be intimidated by medical professionals when you confront them. Remember, they are in business. And remember, so are you. It is your business to get the best care at the lowest cost.

This book will help you do that.

Charles B. Inlander
President
People's Medical Society

We have tried to use male and female pronouns in an egalitarian manner throughout this book. Any imbalance in usage has been in the interests of readability.

CHAPTER 1

Doctors

D octors are the so-called gatekeepers of the medical world.
Through them you enter the worlds of the hospital,
laboratory, and pharmacy. But doctors are also much more. Not
only do they determine the quantity of health care you receive
and set the price, but they're also responsible for the *quality* of
care you receive. Doctors control every aspect and avenue of the
health care delivery system, and for these reasons–and more
personal ones as well–you'll want to develop a good working
relationship with your doctor. Knowing how to interact with a
doctor makes you a smarter consumer, improving your prospects
of getting high quality care. And by working carefully and
assertively with your practitioners, you can greatly lower your
health costs.

But first things first–how do you go about looking for Dr.
Right? The fact of the matter is that most consumers spend more
time selecting a roofer than they do choosing someone to look
after their health. Choosing a doctor isn't easy. It's a process filled
with questions, both for the prospective doctor and for yourself,
but the savvy consumer will realize that the right choice will save
money and perhaps even a life.

Begin your search by getting a few good recommendations
from family members, friends, and neighbors. Word of mouth is
still one of the best methods of finding out which doctors are
taking new patients and what others think of these doctors. The
old adage of "If you want to find a good doctor, ask a nurse" is

probably a good one but not always practical. And don't overlook your present doctor, especially if your relationship with this doctor is ending because he is leaving practice or retiring. Ask him for names of other practitioners to consider. Other sources that may help you find a doctor are:

▶ *Doctor referral services operated by a local medical society (usually county-based).* Not necessarily our first choice, such services will refer only those doctors who are members of the society.

▶ *Hospital-sponsored physician referral services.* Similar to medical society referral services, in this case a local hospital refers you to a list of physicians who are either on their staff or have privileges at their facility. Neither referral service will comment on the specific ability of referred physicians other than to perhaps mention board credentials.

▶ *Newspaper advertisements of doctors announcing the opening of a new practice.* Be wary, however, and ask yourself why the doctor is advertising. To attract patients because she is just out of medical school? Or is in a highly competitive and glutted market? Or has she just moved in from a state where her license was revoked?

▶ *Your company personnel office.* Ask if your company maintains a list of doctors other employees have recommended.

▶ *Your health insurance company.* Check if your insurer has any local doctors to recommend or, in the area of a major problem, it recommends specialists for particular conditions.

▶ *Listings in the telephone directory.* Doctors' names are usually arranged according to practice or specialty, but be aware that just because a doctor says she specializes in a certain area of medicine does not mean the doctor actually took any advanced training in it. A doctor can practice in any specialty area she chooses.

▶ *Senior centers.* Some have referral services.

Here now are some savvy tips for dealing with doctors.

1.
Check for board certification.

Physicians who are board certified have to meet additional training requirements and must pass a rigorous examination administered by a specialty board. Since a large difference in fees between certified and noncertified physicians is unlikely, you may as well go with the doctor who has additional training–*if* he indeed does. Physicians know that consumers are more savvy about credentials, so they're doing everything they can to make themselves look better. So be alert to physicians who play a little game by putting initials after their name. They're counting on your being impressed when you see the initials "B.E." following their name. Don't be; it only means "board eligible."

Another favorite ploy of some physicians is to list themselves as board certified, but fail to tell you in which specialty. You've got to make sure that the physician is board certified in his main field of practice. To check the board-certification status of a physician, call the American Board of Medical Specialties. The group's toll-free number is 800-776-CERT. (When you call, have at hand the physician's full name and his city and state.)

2.
Ask for a get-acquainted visit.

Before seeking the professional services of a new doctor, we suggest that you contact several physicians to determine if they are accepting new patients. If they are, set up a short get-acquainted visit and offer to pay for the time. (According to a recent survey among physicians, the fee for a brief visit is between $22 and $35. Some physicians may not charge you for the time, but always offer to pay; it's one investment that will return dividends.) The purpose of this visit is to find out if you and the doctor see eye to eye on health issues and if her office services are efficient, and to have any of your questions answered *before* you commit to her services. No matter how thorough your doctor-shopping expedition has been, many problems do not arise until the first face-to-face encounter with the practitioner and the office staff.

3.

Check fees in advance.

There is a surprising amount of variation in basic fees, and, indeed, doctors tend not to publish or post their fees for a variety of reasons. The primary one is that they do not have a set fee for a given procedure. (The skeptic would say that the fees doctors charge have nothing to do with their qualifications – they are more likely to be due to the size of the doctor's mortgage or car payment.)

Each time you visit the doctor, ask what the charges will be for the procedures, tests, and treatments the doctor will perform. If the doctor does not know what his fees are, then insist that the person who does know come into the room with you and the doctor.

4.

Negotiate charges and fees.

Most people never think of negotiating with a doctor. Negotiating is something we do with a car dealer or a flea market vendor. The savvy consumer, however, never forgets that medicine is a business – in fact, the biggest business in America – and therefore, normal business practices apply, including negotiation.

Generally, doctors are willing to lower their standard fees for patients with limited incomes or special economic circumstances. Mind you, doctors probably won't readily admit that they negotiate their fees, but in reality they do. Every time a physician signs an insurance agreement, she is permitting someone else to set the price of service. Businesses have also taken actions that force employees to shop for the best price among physicians. By setting maximum reimbursement levels on insurance plans, businesses are telling employees to find the best value. Physicians are well aware of this practice and, because of increased competition, are more willing to adjust their fees in order to get the business.

Here's the strategy: If the quoted fee seems excessively high or is more than you can pay, tell the doctor. Indicate that you feel this is wrong or that you cannot afford such a cost. Ask if the fee can be lowered in your case or if some other payment scheme can be devised. If you have been using the physician for many years, call upon your loyal patronage. Remember, doctors' services are like airline fares: No two people are necessarily paying the same amount for the same class of service to the same destination. And just like the airlines, a doctor's financial security over the long haul is based on your repeat business.

5.
Make it clear to your doctor that all tests must be specifically approved by you before ordering.

Millions of medical tests are performed annually, and Americans and insurers spend billions of dollars for them. Yet many millions of these tests are not necessary, say some experts. And many of the tests aren't very accurate. Others have serious risks and iffy benefits. So you may well wonder—should you have that test? Does your malady really require two or three tests to determine a diagnosis?

The savvy consumer *can* take charge and *can* minimize the risks and costs of unnecessary or excessive testing.

▶ *Ask why you need the test.* Before you agree to any test, ask your doctor what will be done if the test results are abnormal and what will be done if the test results are normal.

▶ *Ask how reliable the test is, what the chance is of a false-positive or false-negative result, and how risks of either can be minimized.* (A false-positive result means that the test shows up positive, or abnormal, but no disease is actually present. A false-negative result means that the test shows up negative, or normal, but you actually have the disease.) Mind you, no test is 100 percent accurate, but you should be told the usefulness and the limits of tests if you are to make an informed decision.

▶ *Find out what alternatives you have if you refuse the test.*

▶ *Ask how much the test will cost.* And don't forget to check with your insurance company prior to undergoing an expensive test to see if it will cover the total cost.

6.
Check if the doctor uses an in-office laboratory.

In-office labs tend to be less expensive, but just as with any commercial laboratory, the test results are only as good as the people and equipment carrying out the test. Furthermore, regulations and standards governing in-office laboratories vary from state to state, and critics of office-based testing point to problems with accuracy, quality and quality control, lack of adequately trained laboratory staff and staff turnover—and incentive to profit through overtesting. Study after study shows small in-office laboratories tend to have a greater variability in test results than do large, regulated labs. Any one of these problems can take a toll on your health and finances.

So be sure to ask your doctor if her lab is inspected and certified. Find out the qualifications of the people working in the lab. What are their credentials? Is anyone a medical technologist, trained in the proper collection and preparation of specimens and the operation of the equipment? How often is the equipment inspected and calibrated, and when was the last time this was done?

7.
Discuss all options before agreeing to tests.

Doctors have come to rely on tests to such an extent that they tend to order them routinely, whether or not they're necessary to confirm a diagnosis. Discuss the necessity of each and every recommended test in detail with your doctor. Consult *The People's Book of Medical Tests,* by David S. Sobel, M.D., and Tom Ferguson, M.D. (New York: Summit Books, 1985) for more information on the test. Unnecessary medical testing, done solely as a defensive measure, costs consumers a whopping $15 billion a year!

Even in the area of testing, negotiation can play an important role. Let's assume the doctor recommends a particular test. Here's how to negotiate whether it is the most appropriate one for your current situation: Begin by asking why this particular test. Ask if there is a more comprehensive test that will answer more questions. Ask the doctor to explain the risks associated as well as matters like pain or time involved with the procedure.

Of course, ask the price and be prepared to pinpoint whether that price is all-inclusive.

When you get all the information, sit down with the doctor and negotiate what you want. Don't be afraid to ask more questions or make decisions that are not necessarily what the doctor might have originally recommended. Make sure this is a give-and-take situation. Ask the doctor, "If I do X, what are my chances that Y will occur?" In other words, come to an agreement.

In 1983 the People's Medical Society created the Code of Practice as a statement we believe each doctor should subscribe to. Ask your doctor to review it and tell you whether he or she will apply it to your care.

THE PEOPLE'S MEDICAL SOCIETY CODE OF PRACTICE

I will assist you in finding information resources, support groups, and health care providers to help you maintain and improve your health. When you seek my care for specific problems, I will abide by the following Code of Practice:

I. *Office Procedures*

1. I will post or provide a printed schedule of my fees for office visits, procedures, tests, and surgery, and provide itemized bills.

2. I will provide certain hours each week when I will be available for nonemergency telephone consultation.

3. I will schedule appointments to allow the necessary time to see you with minimal waiting. I will promptly report test results to you and return phone calls.

4. I will allow and encourage you to bring a friend or relative into the examining room with you.

5. I will facilitate your getting your medical and hospital records, and will provide you with copies of your test results.

continued on next page

THE PEOPLE'S MEDICAL SOCIETY CODE OF PRACTICE
continued

II. Choice in Diagnosis and Treatment

1. I will let you know your prognosis, including whether your condition is terminal or will cause disability or pain, and will explain why I believe further diagnostic activity or treatment is necessary.

2. I will discuss with you diagnostic, treatment, and medication options for your particular problem (including the option of no treatment), and describe in understandable terms the risk of each alternative, the chances of success, the possibility of pain, the effect on your functioning, the number of visits each would entail, and the cost of each alternative.

3. I will describe my qualifications to perform the proposed diagnostic measures or treatments.

4. I will let you know of organizations, support groups, and medical and lay publications that can assist you in understanding, monitoring, and treating your problem.

5. I will not proceed until you are satisfied that you understand the benefits and risks of each alternative and I have your agreement on a particular course of action.

8.

Make it clear to your doctor that all consultations with other physicians must be specifically approved by you prior to ordering.

Especially during periods of hospitalization, you may find yourself being billed for consultations by specialists that you may not even have known took place, much less that you approved. Also check with your insurance company or employee benefits office before agreeing to any consultations; some companies require precertification, which means that the service, the consultation, or even the test must be approved in advance. Failure to get prior approval could reduce your benefit and result in a large out-of-pocket expense for you.

9.
Buy a medical guide to aid you in deciding whether or not to see a doctor.

There are several good home medical guides available that offer clear advice and instructions for determining whether a doctor's care is necessary. These are just a few such guides:

Mayo Clinic Family Health Book, edited by David E. Larson, M.D. (New York: William Morrow, 1990).

Take Care of Yourself: Your Personal Guide to Self-Care and Preventing Illness (4th ed.), Donald M. Vickery, M.D., and James F. Fries, M.D. (Reading, MA: Addison-Wesley, 1989).

The American Medical Association Family Medical Guide (rev. ed.), edited by Jeffrey R. M. Kuntz, M.D., and Asher J. Finkel, M.D. (New York: Random House, 1987).

The American Medical Association Home Medical Advisor, edited by Charles Clayman, M.D., et al. (New York: Random House, 1988).

The Columbia University College of Physicians and Surgeons Complete Home Medical Guide (rev. ed.), edited by Donald F. Tapley, M.D., et al. (New York: Crown, 1989).

The New Good Housekeeping Family Health and Medical Guide (New York: Hearst Books, 1989).

10.
Do not use a specialist as a primary-care physician.

A primary-care physician is one who cares for the whole patient and has not specialized in any one area of the body or condition. Adults have three types of primary-care physicians from which to choose:

▶ *General practitioners.* Though dwindling in numbers, some G.P.'s still practice today.

► *Family practitioners.* Doctors who intend to become F.P.'s take additional training beyond medical school–a three-year residency that covers certain aspects of internal medicine, gynecology, minor surgery, obstetrics, pediatrics, orthopedics, and preventive medicine–and then pass a comprehensive examination.

► *Internists.* Like family practitioners, these doctors complete a three-year residency and must pass a comprehensive examination, but they do not normally take training in pediatrics, orthopedics, and child delivery. Instead they have more advanced training in diagnosis and management of problems involving areas such as the gastrointestinal system, the heart, the kidney, the liver, and the endocrine system.

If you require the care of a specialist for a specific problem (such as a cardiologist for a heart problem), do not ask that person to treat any problems not related to that particular specialty. Not only are a specialist's time and care more expensive, but he may not be the best qualified to deal with problems outside of his specific area of expertise.

11.

Always go to a nonspecialist first— specialists are rarely necessary.

As you can see from the previous item, primary-care physicians are able to treat the vast majority of illnesses, and they will readily refer you to a specialist if necessary. But in the meantime you will have paid less for the care you received. Furthermore, self-referral to a specialist has potential problems. Sure, at some time or another any of us may need a specialist to help discover the cause of a troublesome problem or to manage an uncommon or uncomplicated disease; however, out of the obvious need for experts in fields of medicine has come an overspecialized, fragmented system of medical care. And out of this has sprung the phenomenon of, for example, the orthopedist who sees "the back problem" and not the person as a whole, the urologist who sees "the bladder infection" and not the person's complete medical condition, and so on. Specialization profoundly influences the way medicine is practiced. Too often patients are referred from doctor to doctor to be reassured that nothing is wrong with the organ system of the doctor's field of interest or specialty.

Self-refer only if you must and if you feel that you, alone or preferably with an advocate (a friend or relative) by your side, can maintain control over any decisions regarding tests, procedures, and so on. But first determine what type of specialist you need, or even if you need one. Furthermore, if you belong to a health maintenance organization (HMO) or preferred provider organization (PPO) and decide to see a specialist *first*—in short, self-refer, a practice that HMOs and PPOs frown upon—you could be responsible for the entire cost of the visit.

WHAT IS A SPECIALIST?

A specialist is a doctor who concentrates on a specific body system, age group, or disorder. After obtaining an M.D. (Doctor of Medicine) or D.O. (Doctor of Osteopathy) degree, a doctor then undergoes two to three years of supervised specialty training (called a *residency*). Many specialists also take one or more years of additional training (called a *fellowship*) in a specific area of their specialty (called a *subspecialty*).

How can you tell if a doctor is a trained specialist? A doctor who has taken extra training in his or her field often chooses to become board certified. In addition to the extra training, the doctor must pass a rigorous examination administered by a specialty board, a national board of professionals in that specialty field. A doctor who passes the board examination is given the status of *Diplomate*. Plus, most board-certified doctors become members of their medical specialty societies, and any doctor who meets the full requirements for membership is called a *Fellow* of the society and may use the designation. For instance, the title "FACOG" after a doctor's name denotes that he or she is a Fellow of the American College of Obstetricians and Gynecologists.

12.
Demand itemized bills.

Itemized bills are always a good idea because they let you know exactly what you are paying for and help you determine whether you are being billed for a service you did not receive. Sometimes even an itemized bill doesn't give you enough information to make such determinations. Hospitals and doctors use esoteric codes; if such codes appear on your statement, without explanation, contact the business office and ask for a statement in plain English. If you are still not clear about a charge, or have a dispute, ask your doctor to verify that a particular service, test, or product was ordered for your care.

13.
Use ambulatory care centers (or walk-in/walk-out centers) rather than hospital emergency rooms if your doctor is not available.

Anytime you feel you need a doctor's care, you should call your doctor first. But if your doctor is not available, an ambulatory care center (sometimes called urgicenter or emergicenter) is usually less expensive and less time-consuming than a hospital emergency room. Such facilities—either independent clinics or affiliated with hospitals—offer basic medical care on a walk-in basis for 12 or even 24 hours of the day, rather than only during traditional office hours. The mission in most primary/emergency/ urgent care centers is to treat minor injuries or short-term illnesses and provide immediate treatment for routine problems: for example, cuts, sprains, dislocated or broken bones, sore throats, and earaches.

14.
Get a second opinion.

First isn't always best. It's odd, though—people are willing, even eager, to ask for seconds on just about everything, except medical diagnoses. It is always a good idea, for your health as well as your pocketbook, to get a second opinion on any invasive procedure your doctor recommends, whether diagnostic or surgical. Review the information on benefits in your insurance plan concerning when a second opinion is required and covered. Some companies require a second opinion for all elective procedures; however, if you forgo the second opinion, you may discover that your coverage has been reduced by half. But regardless of who pays, it is always smart to get a second opinion, especially if a trip to the hospital looms in your near future. Studies show that there is often substantial disagreement about diagnoses and treatment options.

15.
Get more than two opinions when the first two disagree.

If the second opinion does not agree with the first, it is often a good idea to get a third or even fourth opinion. What you are looking for is a consensus among practitioners, which allows you to make an informed decision about the best course of action. And thorough investigation on your part is the surest way to avoid unnecessary treatment and to save money in the long run.

16.
Get independent second opinions. Don't rely on a second opinion referral from your own doctor.

A lot of second opinion doctors recommended by first opinion doctors turn out to be professional ditto marks and not all that valuable in terms of independent judgments. This is true in part because surgeons are the doctors most often asked for second opinions, and they're hardly predisposed to recommend sheathing the knife. It's also true that doctors often refer patients to other doctors for nonmedical reasons, such as the fact that they're golf buddies or "I owe him a favor." You are less likely to get an impartial, objective second opinion from your doctor's friend or close colleague. In addition, chances are that your doctor will call and discuss your case with the person to whom he referred you, and the second opinion will be made before the second doctor has a chance to examine you.

To find your own physician for a second opinion, start by contacting your insurance company and requesting a list of physicians who participate in second opinion programs. Do the same with your employer's benefits manager and your union, if you're a union member. Check the *Directory of Medical Specialists* in your local library's reference section. Ask friends who might have had similar conditions what doctor they used. The point is—shop around to find the most objective and competent practitioner available.

17.
Explore the non-M.D. providers when possible.

Basic health care can often be provided competently, safely and less expensively by non-M.D.'s such as optometrists, podiatrists, chiropractors, audiologists, physician assistants, nurse-midwives, and nurse practitioners. A quick glance through the medical services section of the *Dictionary of Occupational Titles* will find hundreds of professional occupations concerned with treating and caring for sick and injured people. Some of these practitioners support and complement the services of doctors and dentists, while others practice independently, depending upon the laws of the particular state in which they are licensed.

These so-called limited license providers can save you money if used properly. As a savvy consumer, you should always check their credentials to make certain they are properly licensed or certified—especially important if your insurance plan requires that all non-M.D. providers must be licensed or certified in accordance with the laws of your state.

18.
Call ahead to see if the doctor is running on time.

Just as the savvy traveler calls the airport to see if a flight is on schedule, you can save a lot of time (and money, if you must take time off from work) if you call your doctor's office and ask whether appointments are running on schedule. And if you see a doctor regularly, ask the receptionist to call you if appointments are running late. This allows you to either adjust your schedule or change the appointment.

19.
Send the doctor a bill if she keeps you waiting for more than 30 minutes.

The idea that patients actually bill doctors for waiting time is no longer a novelty. (Not long ago a savvy Florida man sued his doctor for excessive waiting and won!) Medical practice management experts have taken note of this and are now telling doctors that they had better get used to it. One expert told a doctor to adjust the patient's bill for the next office visit. In short, value your time and remember that you have lost not only the time in the waiting room, but also the time it took you to get there and back.

20.
Use a doctor with separate waiting rooms for sick and well visits.

More and more doctors are offering this convenience, particularly for children. Doctors' offices are prime places to pick up illnesses, and more illnesses mean more money. How smart is it to pay to see a doctor, then pay again for something you "caught" in the waiting room? If your doctor doesn't provide such a service, recommend he do so.

21.
Make sure the doctor accepts your insurance coverage.

Always confirm, at the time you make the appointment, that the doctor accepts the health insurance that you carry *and* will accept your insurance reimbursement as "payment in full," less required copayments or deductibles. These three little words can lead to trouble if you and your doctor's billing staff are using the same words but speaking a different language. A simple misunderstanding here can lead to balance billing, the practice of billing the patient for the difference between the doctor's usual charge and the amount paid by the insurance company. Clarify these points ahead of time.

22.
Get a job in a hospital.

It may sound facetious, but it really can be a money saver. Hospitals often give employees free services—although in recent years some hospitals have modified their benefits plans to include deductibles.

23.
Make sure a family member becomes a doctor.

But don't pay for the relative's education!

24.
Don't offhandedly substitute an emergency room for your doctor.

Never go to an emergency room (except in absolute emergencies) unless you at least try to contact your doctor first. If your doctor does not make provisions for seeing people at relatively short notice during office hours, find another doctor. To avoid out-of-pocket expenses, check your insurance coverage concerning when ER visits are covered and when not. Another reason for avoiding the ER, if possible, is what you may encounter there. Less than desirable conditions and possibly a long wait. Some reports indicate that a wait of seven to 10 hours is not that unusual in certain cities and regions; so such a visit not only costs you more money, but it also wastes your valuable time.

If you are enrolled in a health maintenance organization (HMO), ideally your HMO will want you to use its emergency center or an affiliated hospital's emergency room for immediate treatment. However, as you know, not every emergency situation is so strategically and conveniently orchestrated. Find out your HMO's rules in the event you seek emergency care during night and weekend hours or away from home, as well as its rule should your calls to your primary-care physician go unanswered. Be smart and find out *ahead* of the time you *really* need this information.

25.
Seek telephone advice from your doctor whenever possible.

Most doctors are happy to answer questions and provide advice over the phone about medication, reactions to treatment, or recurring health problems. Ever since the People's Medical Society promoted the use of set-aside telephone hours in our physician Code of Practice (see pages 19 and 20), the concept has been catching on. You can save a considerable amount of money and perhaps unnecessary anguish by avoiding office visits for simple medical advice.

26.
Get to know your doctor's office staff.

Many problems can be solved and questions answered by a doctor's office staff, and, frankly, it's just smart to make yourself known to the people who control really important aspects of a medical practice. Patients are generally not charged for brief consultations with the office nurse – by phone or in person.

27.
Demand that the doctor accept Medicare payments on assignment.

Most doctors are willing to accept Medicare on assignment – which means that you will not be required to pay more than your 20 percent copayment – on a case-by-case basis. If your doctor is hesitant about accepting assignment, remind her that Medicare's new fee schedule will mean better and faster reimbursement. If your doctor refuses, find another doctor.

If you can't find another doctor, you can still save money on nonparticipating physicians (those docs who have not agreed to accept the Medicare-approved amounts as payments in full) thanks to limits on balance billing. New Medicare regulations limit the maximum payment to nonparticipating physicians, so they can't bill you for the full difference between the Medicare-approved amount and their regular fee if it exceeds 120 percent (in 1992) or 115 percent (in 1993).

28.
Read about your condition.

You will be able to make savvy, more informed decisions about your treatment—and avoid possibly unnecessary tests and procedures—if you know a lot about your condition and ask the logical and informed questions. Only then will you be able to be a major partner in making your health decisions. And don't neglect to take advantage of a free service right there in your own community: your local public library. If you have not discovered the resources, ingenuity, and helpfulness that a reference librarian has to offer, then by all means do so. Even if you live in a small community with a modest library, one with a limited catalog of medical and health books, there's always interlibrary loan. In addition, hospitals will often let you use their medical libraries.

29.
Say "No" if you do not understand, and ask questions until you do.

Never submit to a test, treatment, or procedure that you do not fully understand. You should be able to answer four questions about any treatment you doctor recommends:

1. What is the purpose of this test/procedure/medication?
2. How will it help my condition?

3. Are there less costly, and equally as safe, alternatives to what you propose?

4. What are the possible side effects, and what is the probability that one or more will occur?

Don't be intimidated by comments such as "Who's the doctor here?" or "It's to make you better." Every unnecessary test or procedure costs you money, not to mention time and possible discomfort.

30.
Demand a full justification of any tests or procedures.

Just as in number 29, you can make an informed decision about your doctor's recommendations only if you understand them and you know why a particular treatment is preferable to others.

31.
Look for free or low-priced community services.

Many communities offer flu shots, immunizations, simple screening tests, cholesterol screening, occult blood screening, and certain other health-related services through the county health department. Also visit health fairs in your area to learn more about services that are available in your community at no, or nominal, cost.

32.
Always ask if it is possible to use previous X rays rather than take new ones.

Doctors often order X rays because they do not know that previous X rays exist. Keep a complete record of X rays—what type, when, how many different exposures—and request that X rays be promptly sent to a new doctor. Even simple X rays are expensive (and can be dangerous), so they should be taken only if absolutely necessary.

33.
Avoid mobile X-ray units.

Mobile X-ray units often use miniature films that require a greater X-ray exposure. Also, these mobile units are used primarily for chest screening for tuberculosis, which is usually unnecessary.

34.
If you are a woman and under 50, consult your physician about the need for routine mammography.

In light of recent headlines on breast cancer rates, the savvy medical consumer who's a woman undoubtedly is wondering what to do and when. There is great debate among medical experts about when routine mammography is useful to begin. The benefits of mammography for women between the ages of 50 and 65 seem to be clear; studies done around the world show that regular screening mammograms can cut the death rate from breast cancer by 30 percent or more in these women. But among women between the ages of 40 and 49 or younger, the benefit of regular screening mammograms is much less clear, and the risk of undergoing unnecessary treatment (or not getting treatment you need) because of inaccurate results is much greater.

The American Cancer Society and the National Cancer Institute (along with nine other medical organizations, four of them professional radiology groups) endorse screening mammograms at one- or two-year intervals for women between the ages of 40 and 49. Two large professional groups, the American College of Surgeons and the American College of Physicians, have declined to recommend routine mammography screening for women 40 to 49 years old. And a panel of experts assembled by the U.S. Department of Health and Human Services recently concluded that mammography screening for women under 50 should be done only when there is a family history of the disease.

You should also remember that insurance companies usually will not reimburse for diagnostic tests that aren't medically necessary. This means that any such expense comes out of your pocket. In any case, be sure to discuss mammography thoroughly with your doctor.

35.
Avoid fluoroscopy if an ordinary X ray can do the job.

Fluoroscopy exposes you to much more X-ray radiation and, therefore, should never be used if a simple X ray will serve. Overkill on tests is a tendency many doctors have—and it's your wallet (and health) that suffers.

36.
Question routine preemployment X rays.

People whose jobs will require them to handle food or work with people are often required to be screened for tuberculosis by state laws. Nowadays there are perfectly acceptable non-X-ray tests to screen for tuberculosis that do not require radiation, so resist a chest X ray for this purpose.

37.
Refuse routine dental X rays.

Again, X-ray examinations are expensive and possibly dangerous, so you should never agree to them unless they are necessary to diagnose a problem.

38.
If you change dentists or go to a dental specialist, take your dental X rays with you.

There is no reason to submit to an additional set of X rays by a new dentist if you have had X rays fairly recently done. Just take your old ones along with you.

39.

Following three or more normal Pap smears one year apart, the Pap test may be performed less frequently at the discretion of your physician.

In 1988 the American Cancer Society adopted this policy, similar to that endorsed by the American College of Obstetricians and Gynecologists, the National Cancer Institute, and the American Medical Association. What's a good time interval? A recent study by researchers at the University of Washington in Seattle suggests that going more than two years without a Pap smear increases your risk of developing cervical cancer.

40.

Have routine screening tests done by non-M.D.'s.

In many cases routine screening tests can be done just as accurately by non-M.D.'s—for example, nurse-midwives in the case of Pap smears. It is usually more expensive to take the time of a fully qualified physician to perform simple tests than to use a nurse or other non-M.D.

CHAPTER 2

Drugs

You don't need to be an economist to know that the cost of prescription drugs has gone through the roof. In the 1980s inflation rose 58 percent, while in the same decade drug prices increased a whopping 152 percent. A prescription that cost $20 in 1980 now costs $53.76. And at that rate, it will cost $77.06 in 1995 and $120.88 in 2000.

What is a bitter pill for you, the consumer, to swallow is, on the other hand, a prescription for profit for the drug manufacturing industry. A 1991 report of the U.S. Senate Special Committee on Aging stated that while the average Fortune 500 industry in this country had an average profitability of 4.6 percent in 1990, the average profitability of the top 10 drug companies more than tripled that amount: 15.5 percent.

How can you stay on the winning side in this multibillion-dollar-a-year industry? Be savvy and protect yourself from the outrageous price increases. Think smart and know where to go to find out whether the drug your doctor prescribes for you is the best, most efficacious medication for your condition. Granted, in a nation that fills approximately 1.6 billion prescriptions each year and has some 2,500 drugs on the market, even the wisest of medical consumers cannot become familiar with the names of all the available prescription and over-the-counter medications. But the winning strategy is to arm yourself with information on as many "fronts" as you can: everything from choosing the best pharmacist and comparison-shopping for brand name, generic, and over-the-counter drugs to avoiding costly and potentially dangerous medication errors.

41.
Know your pharmacist.

A pharmacist can be an invaluable resource for information regarding drugs—any interactions to be aware of, alternative forms of the same drug (i.e., liquid or pills), and less expensive alternatives. You see, more than a pill counter, the pharmacist is the most readily accessible health care professional most of us have—a highly trained drug expert who probably knows more than your own physician about the relative benefits and risks of various drugs. With today's medications more complex and, in some cases, more potent, and with drug prescribing on the increase, the savvy medical consumer will find a competent and communicative pharmacist. It's also smart to talk with your pharmacist, for the better she knows you, the more she will be able to help.

WHAT A GOOD PHARMACIST DOES: A CHECKLIST

✔ Does more than merely read a doctor's prescription, fill it, label it, and charge for it.

✔ Keeps important family medication records called patient medication profiles, and uses them to prevent allergic reactions to drugs, dangerous interactions, duplicate medications, and drug abuse.

✔ Advises how to use prescription and nonprescription medication; how and when to take it; what the possible side effects are; what the shelf life is; how to store the medication; and whether there is potential for dangerous interactions with foods and/or other medications.

✔ Answers your questions about the staggering variety of medicines, remedies, tonics, pills, elixirs, lotions, salves, capsules, and powders on the market.

✔ Advises you, when necessary, to seek a medical practitioner's help.

42.
Shop around for prescription prices.

Prescription drug prices vary about as much as a nervous stock market, and it's no secret that drug companies have raised their prices to wholesalers. So now, more than ever, you've got to become a determined shopper. On any given day you may be able to find better prices for the medications you need. Contact the large chain pharmacies first since they usually offer better discounts because of their bulk-buying practices. This, however, is not to say that a local pharmacy may not have a better price on a particular drug. Even if you have a prescription plan where you work, shopping for the lowest drug price is important, especially if you have a copayment based on a percentage of the total cost of the prescription.

43.
Buy generic prescription drugs whenever possible.

A generic drug (the name of which is usually a condensed version of the drug's original chemical name) is one whose active ingredients duplicate those of the brand name product. While a generic does not have to be the same size, shape, or color of the brand name, by law it does have to be bioequivalent, determined by how much of the drug is absorbed into the bloodstream and how quickly absorption takes place. A generic cannot differ from the pioneer drug by more than 20 percent in either the speed or amount of absorption.

So much for what it is, now why buy? On the average, generic drugs are 30 percent cheaper than their brand name cousins — even 50 to 70 percent cheaper than the more expensive medicines. Mind you, the generic is *usually* cheaper than the brand name drug, but always check with your doctor or pharmacist to determine whether a generic form of the drug you need is available, safe, and less expensive. Also, since laws vary across the country, ask what your state's law is concerning the substitution of generic for brand name drugs. The generic pharmaceutical industry can provide you with more information on generic drugs and their use. For a copy of their free guide, contact:

Generic Pharmaceutical Industry Association
200 Madison Avenue, Suite 2402
New York, NY 10016

10 OF THE MOST COMMONLY PRESCRIBED DRUGS AND THEIR GENERIC VERSIONS

Brand Name/Generic Name	Prescribed For
Amoxil/amoxicillin	antibiotic
Lanoxin/digoxin	heart
Zantac/ranitidine hydrochloride	ulcer
Premarin/conjugated estrogens	hormone
Xanax/alprazolam	anxiety
Dyazide/hydrochlorothiazide, triamterene	high blood pressure
Cardizem/diltiazem hydrochloride	heart
Tenormin/atenolol	heart
Naprosyn/naproxen	arthritis
Tagamet/cimetidine	ulcer

44.
Buy store-brand over-the-counter, or nonprescription, drugs whenever possible.

Many pharmacies and some grocery store chains purchase over-the-counter (OTC) drugs in bulk and package them under their own store's brand name or label. By reading labels you can compare prices on brand name items to the less expensive, but identical, store-brand item. But first, before you plunk down your cash for an OTC remedy with possibly questionable effectiveness, find out if a formerly prescription-only drug is available without a prescription. As the Food and Drug Administration (FDA) lifts the prescription-only restriction from many products, most notably decongestants and hydrocortisone,

over-the-counter medications become available to treat the same
symptoms that prescription drugs treat. The effectiveness of
these medications has been proven, and it makes sense to spend
your money for these products.

Indeed, Americans treat their ailments without professional
help and often with nonprescription medicines some 60 percent
of the time, according to an *American Pharmacy* article. Before
you self-medicate, however, talk with your doctor or pharmacist
about similar over-the-counter drugs. Remember, too, that some
nonprescription drugs are as strong as the medications your doctor
prescribes. As for the FDA's stamp of approval or the agency's
eagerness to remove a suspect drug from the market, let's just say
that ineffective and marginally effective drugs do exist.

A word of warning, though: The savvy medical consumer
makes a point of consulting a pharmacist or physician before
buying any OTC preparations for babies, young children, elderly
or debilitated persons, or pregnant or breast-feeding women.

45.
Buy single-ingredient over-the-counter drugs.

Many over-the-counter drugs are preparations of several drugs,
for example a "cold" medication that combines an antihistamine
with a decongestant. It is less expensive to purchase a decongestant and an antihistamine separately—because often you will
need only one of these to treat your symptoms and because
mixtures can be more expensive.

Here are a few other wise strategies for selecting the best OTCs
and getting the most for your money:

► Find out the risks or side effects of any OTC you're
considering buying and taking.

► Ask about potentially dangerous interactions between
over-the-counter medications and any prescription drugs you
may be taking. Common products such as nose drops, antacids,
and aspirin can interfere with the actions and effectiveness of
prescription drugs.

► Go over with your pharmacist the label instructions of any
medication so that you can be sure you're taking it wisely and

appropriately—especially if you're taking drug preparations in forms you do not normally use or fully understand: suppositories or prolonged-release tablets, for instance.

46.
Break the code.

What we are talking about is shorthand code that doctors, pharmacists, and nurses share as part of a long tradition of cryptic communication that excludes consumers. Particularly prominent are the medical abbreviations that are scrawled across prescription forms. Fortunately for the smart medical consumer, translating those enigmatic terms into everyday language is not difficult. Here's a list of some Latin directions to pharmacists and common abbreviations that turn up frequently on prescription sheets (some doctors may use variations of these symbols):

Abbreviation (on prescription)	English meaning
ad lib.	as needed
a.c.	before meals
p.c.	after meals
b.i.d.	twice a day
t.i.d.	three times a day
q.i.d.	four times a day
h.s.	at bedtime
p.o.	orally (by mouth)
q.4h	every four hours
q.8h	every eight hours
ut dict.	as directed by doctor
OD	right eye (drops)
OS	left eye (drops)
OU	both eyes (drops)

47.
Ask for an initial one to two days' supply of any new prescription to check for side effects.

Since the possibility exists for an adverse reaction to *any* medication, you will save your health and money if you initially request only one to two days' supply of a new prescription. You can pick up the remainder of the prescription (and pay for it) the next day if no adverse reaction occurs.

48.
Ask your doctor for free samples.

Physicians regularly receive free samples of prescription and over-the-counter medications from pharmaceutical company representatives. Again, it's wise to initially stockpile only a few days' worth of an unknown drug until you are sure that you and it are compatible. Think of it as a test drive, something any savvy consumer would do first.

49.
Purchase drugs directly from your doctor.

Let us first say that the practice called physician dispensing is not without its critics; indeed, the entire issue has raised quite a hue and cry in the prescription drug industry lately–in part because it upsets the so-called natural order of business wherein doctors prescribe and pharmacists dispense. The pharmacists call it an encroachment on their territory and a source of potential harm to consumers. Meanwhile the doctors call it good for their patients and bottom-line smart for their incomes.

What has made this a growth industry is a relatively new business called "repackaging": Companies (called repackagers) buy drugs in bulk at wholesale costs from drug manufacturers, then resell to doctors in convenient, safety-sealed containers, ready for on-the-spot dispensing to their patients.

Frankly, the answer to the question "Is physician dispensing a patient convenience or exploitation?" has more to do with the individual physician than with the practice as a whole. So the savvy medical consumer will get all the facts before buying and taking any prescription drug dispensed by her physician:

▶ Compare the doctor's prices with those of area drug-stores to determine whether there is an economic advantage to the consumer.

▶ Verify if anyone in the doctor's office assures that the drugs dispensed are the right ones, the dosages correct, and the directions clear, complete, and accurate. (After all, physician dispensing sidesteps the highly trained drug expert, the pharmacist.)

50.
Purchase in bulk, when appropriate.

Although individuals cannot buy drugs directly from wholesalers, bulk purchasing is a way you can purchase your medications in larger quantities. If you're taking a certain medication for an extended period of time, have your physician write the prescription for a six-month or longer supply, as opposed to six refills. Some pharmacists may be wary if you ask for your six refills all at once, and your state's pharmacy laws may prohibit such dispensing. That's why it's better to have your physician write in the number of pills—such as 200 or 250—then you can discuss bulk purchases with the pharmacist.

51.
Investigate purchasing by mail order.

The cost savings of doing such, according to the industry's trade organization, range anywhere from 5 to 40 percent off prices at your local pharmacy. The American Association of Retired Persons offers a full-service mail-order pharmacy to members, a program that generally has lower prices than regular pharmacies. Other mail-order businesses offer more specialized medications such as homeopathic remedies and vitamin and mineral supplements. Just make sure that prices are indeed lower before purchasing by mail.

52.
Ask about any available discount.

Many, if not most, pharmacies offer senior citizen discounts. Infants' and children's discounts are also available in some pharmacies. Ask the pharmacist for details.

53.
Purchase a prescription plan.

Most group health insurance policies offer prescription coverage for a small additional premium. Ask if your plan offers this additional coverage as an option.

54.
Keep a patient medication profile on yourself (or make sure someone else is doing so).

No doubt about it—someone should be keeping a medication profile on you, indeed on everyone in your household. It's a system that monitors all the drugs you are taking, in hopes of avoiding medication errors. Actually, the logical site for the profile is your pharmacy. The American Pharmaceutical Association recommends that a patient medication profile contain the following information:

▶ Your name, address, and phone number.

▶ Your and your family's birthdays, so that the pharmacist can check whether the dosage is appropriate to the age of the user.

▶ Any allergies, reactions, or adverse effects you've demonstrated.

▶ A concise health history, including any conditions or diseases that would preclude the use of certain drugs.

▶ The over-the-counter, or nonprescription, medicines you take.

▶ The date and number of each prescription filled for you, the name of the drug, its dosage and strength, quantity, directions for use, and price.

▶ The prescriber and dispenser of every medication you take.

55.
Properly store drugs.

Most drug items need to be kept fresh, just as many food products do, with cool, dry conditions best for preserving them. True, some people, especially those who might in an emergency need to get to their medications at a moment's notice, like to keep multiple vials of their prescription drugs stashed away–in the kitchen, in the bedroom, in the workshop, or even in the car. But tossing pills in with the maps and owner's manual is a prescription for trouble–and meltdown. Ask your pharmacist how to store the drugs you are purchasing.

56.
Guard against overmedication.

It's a fact that drug overdosing occurs in many hospitals' pediatric wards and nurseries. The dosages–some as much as 10 times greater than prescribed–are the result of misplaced decimal points and sloppy computational skills of nurses and doctors who do not understand the appropriate doses for different age groups. But that's not all. Various reports have pointed out that drug overdosing occurs with the low-weight elderly. Not only are doctors failing to adjust doses for body weight in many cases, but they often also do not take into account the ages of the patients. The operative physiologic fact here is that the older you get, the longer it takes for drugs to clear out of your system, so dosages must be adjusted accordingly.

It just makes sense, doesn't it, that correct dosages vary among people just as their ages and weights vary? If a savvy medical consumer knows this, shouldn't a doctor? Well, the problem, according to one study, is that doctors prescribe "by habit, with little adjustment for individual patients." So the next time your doctor writes a prescription for you, ask her to double-check your weight and age against the recommended standard dosage for that medication. It may mean a double-savvy whammy: You'll save money if the effective drug dose is less, and you'll increase your margin of safety for dose-related side effects.

57.
Purchase drugs from your HMO pharmacy.

If you are a member of a health maintenance organization (HMO), find out if it has an in-house pharmacy. HMO pharmacies often sell drugs to members at wholesale cost or slightly above.

58.
Consult drug reference books.

To learn more about the medications that are prescribed for you and your family, consult a drug reference guide. You'll find them in libraries as well as pharmacies. A good guide will list the medication by class—such as an antidiabetic or a calcium channel blocker—by chemical or generic name, and by brand name. There should also be a section in which the medication is described and the condition(s) given for which the medication may be prescribed. Additional sections usually discuss how to use the medication; when not to use it in conjunction with other medications; and what the side effects and contraindications (reasons you shouldn't use the medication) are.

Two good reference guides are the *Physician's Desk Reference* and *The Complete Drug Reference,* the latter published by Consumer Reports Books. A reference librarian can help you locate other sources of prescription drug information. Clearly, the best time to find out that a drug may not be appropriate for you is before you have gone to the expense of having the prescription filled.

59.
Consult consumer buying guides to drugs.

Buying guides to drugs, written especially for consumers, are available in most libraries. In addition to giving you information about specific medications, they also point out which drugs are the most effective and which drugs are not effective. Using the most effective drug for a given condition is ultimately cheaper. Some guides you may want to look for are:

Fifty Plus: The Graedons' People's Pharmacy for Older Adults, Joe and Teresa Graedon (New York: Bantam Books, 1988).

The New People's Pharmacy Book: Drug Breakthroughs for the 1980s, Joe Graedon (New York: Bantam Books, 1985).

Worst Pills, Best Pills, Sidney Wolfe, M.D., et al., (Washington, DC: Public Citizen Health Research Group, 1988).

CHAPTER 3

Hospitals

Where you get your medical care is as important as who provides it. The backdrop not only dictates what treatment you get or do not get, but it makes a *big* difference in how much you pay.

You don't have to be a cost accountant to realize that certain health care settings are more expensive than others, with hospital-based care the steepest. One night in a hospital costs an average of $297 or a total of $2,138 for an average stay (December 1991 figures). And that covers only the room and meals; when drugs, medical tests, and other charges are factored in, the daily cost climbs sharply to $900. In terms of national impact, the dollars and cents quickly add up. In 1991, $256 billion was spent for hospital care. That amounts to $1,024 for every man, woman, and child in the country.

Dollar figures like these are enough to convince most people to reduce the time spent in the hospital, if not completely eliminate hospitalization in favor of another setting. But if you must go in, pay close attention to procedures and medications ordered by your physician, and make sure you know what has been ordered and that you are fully informed of the whys and wherefores. Further, if you must go in, it stands to reason that a close scrutiny of the entire process, from preadmission talks with your doctor, to admission, and on to discharge, has the potential to save you money *and* gets you intimately involved in important decisions about your health and welfare.

Speak up whenever you find something is not what you have been told. Be on the lookout for errors in medications, procedures, and the like that can end up costing you extra days in the hospital, as well as extra money from your pocket.

Using even one of the following money-saving hints will save you *at least* the price of this book. And that's just savvy personal finance!

60.
Don't go unless absolutely necessary.

An unnecessary stay threatens far more than your wallet, as if money alone weren't enough to quibble over the necessity of hospitalization. Hospitals can be hazardous to your health. While in the hospital you are at risk of piling up mounds of charges for procedures and tests, but you are also at risk of acquiring a condition you did not have when you went in. That happens to one out of every five hospital patients, and these conditions not only require additional treatment at additional cost, but they can be deadly as well. One of these so-called iatrogenic (literally, doctor-produced) conditions–nosocomial infection–is produced by microorganisms that dwell with relative impunity in hospitals. Most develop at least 72 hours after admission, which means that some may not become manifest until after discharge.

You could describe nosocomial infections as expensive souvenirs of your hospital stay. And close to one out of every 10 patients admitted to a hospital acquires one of these nasty, and often preventable, souvenirs. It is estimated that the recovery time necessary to combat a nosocomial infection is about four extra days of stay. Expensive as it is–experts estimate that it adds, at a minimum, $2.5 billion to America's medical bill–nosocomial infections can also be deadly souvenirs: Some tallies of infection-related deaths run as high as 100,000 (other estimates are even higher, 300,000 or so) a year.

What does the savvy medical consumer do, however, who needs a particular medical procedure? If you require a surgical procedure, you may be able to avoid the hospital entirely if the surgery can be done on an outpatient basis–you're in by around

9 a.m. and out by 5 p.m. or so. Ask your physician about this option. Outpatient surgery is usually less expensive than inpatient surgery, and you lessen the risk of picking up a nasty germ while in the hospital. In fact, your insurance plan or your employer may require you to investigate outpatient surgery first.

There's also the matter of copayment, that cost-sharing requirement in many insurance policies in which you assume a portion or percentage of the cost of covered services. If your copayment is 20 percent on inpatient services and only 10 percent on outpatient services–a not unlikely scenario–it's to your advantage to select the outpatient setting.

61.
Make sure hospital personnel wash their hands before touching you.

Of all the potentially protective measures you can take (or insist that your caregivers take), this one merits its own individual mention. Why? Well, because most of the hospital-acquired infections are gotten from the contaminated hands of doctors, nurses, and other hospital personnel. The Institute for Child Health Policy and others report that many hospital workers who come in direct contact with patients don't take the time, or are not concerned enough, to perform the simplest and best known of precautionary actions. And doctors are among the worst offenders. You can greatly lower your chances of catching such an infection–and paying for its treatment–simply by refusing to allow hospital personnel to care for you until they have washed their hands.

62.
Protect yourself from nosocomial infections.

There is no surefire defense for you if the rest of the hospital is a vast and bubbling breeding ground. So the first step is to try to gain admission to a hospital that has a good nosocomial record. Ask your doctor about it. Contact your local department of health. Ask the hospital directly, but be on your guard if the hospital paints too rosy a picture. That may mean that the staff is not properly surveying the facility's infection rate, or not surveying at all.

The other line of defense is to be informed. Remember, a savvy medical consumer is armed with information. Know the work areas of the hospital where you are at higher risk:

▶ *Hemodialysis unit.* The equipment here can be a source of hepatitis B, a virulent organism that is difficult to destroy.

▶ *Intensive care unit.* Usually occupied by patients who are extremely weak and thus susceptible to infection, this unit is operated under emergency measures that often have to forsake pristine sanitary procedures in order to save a life.

▶ *Infant nursery.*

▶ *Operating room.*

Nosocomial infections can also pass to patients via the procedural chain of the food services department, due to any one or more factors – nearly all of them with their roots in human error. And a myriad of studies also point to other work areas in the hospital that, because of persistently poor and unprofessional hygiene practices, are breeding grounds, too: the central service department (the unit responsible for processing, storing, and dispensing hospital supplies); the pharmacy; the laundry; the laboratory (where, more than one story goes, workers have to be admonished not to keep their lunches in the same refrigerators as the ones that contain serum or other specimens).

63.
Assert yourself.

While it is true that one-third of all infections treated in hospitals are nosocomial infections, it is also estimated that as many as half are preventable. The savvy medical consumer is, where necessary, assertive. Here are some actions you can take while in the hospital:

▶ If your roommate becomes infected, or if you are concerned that what he or she has could possibly be transmitted to you via the air or through the use of a common bathroom, ask your doctor or the staff nurse-epidemiologist about your risks. Change your room at once if there is any chance you might become infected, because once you are infected it is too late.

► If you are undergoing surgery or a procedure that requires the removal of hair, refuse to be shaven the night before surgery. One study indicates that among people shaved the day prior to their operations, the nosocomial infection rate is 5.6 percent. Chemical depilatories reduce the rate to just 0.6 percent. Using barber clippers to remove hair the morning of surgery yields a low infection rate, too.

► Question whether shaving or clipping is necessary at all. Maybe not—and especially when it comes to ob-gyn situations. Removing hair before vaginal delivery or surgery in that area is probably uncalled for, because the old idea that hair creates a climate for infection is unsubstantiated by clinical studies.

► Have nurses regularly check the drainage of urinary catheters to help maintain cleanliness.

64.
If you deliver your baby in the hospital, get him or her out of there as soon as possible.

Although this advice is somewhat tongue-in-cheek, there is a valid reason for concern. Birthing in hospitals exposes infants to the full range of hospital-acquired infections to which adults are exposed. Upper-respiratory and "staph" infections are common in hospital nurseries. And, aside from the worry you will expend, you are required to pay for the care required to treat these infections.

65.
Refuse admission tests that are not pertinent to your illness or the reason for your hospitalization.

Most hospitals routinely require a variety of blood and urine tests and an X ray upon admission, whatever your age and physical health and whether or not you need them. The American College of Radiology has urged that chest X rays be eliminated as a routine procedure for hospital admissions, tuberculosis screening, and preemployment physicals, and as a general rule it's good to avoid X rays unless absolutely necessary because of the dangers associated with excessive radiation. It is in the best interest of your physical and financial health to refuse unnecessary routine testing.

66.
Use outpatient services.

Many invasive diagnostic tests and simple surgeries can be done on an outpatient basis, an arrangement whereby you arrive in the morning for the procedure and are back home again in the after-noon or evening. As an outpatient you are not officially admitted as an inpatient to the hospital, but you receive hospital care (for example, laboratory work and X rays) without occupying a hospital bed or without receiving room, board, or general nursing care. The growth in outpatient care has been so phenomenal that more and more insurance companies are requiring that certain procedures be done on an outpatient basis—mainly because of the cost savings associated with that setting versus inpatient care. Make sure that you know the requirements and limitations of your insurance coverage; otherwise you may end up paying substantial out-of-pocket costs. Remember, the less time you spend in the hospital, generally the cheaper it will be—and as we discussed before, the less likely you are to acquire a nosocomial infection.

67.
Don't stay overnight for diagnostic tests.

Most diagnostic tests can be done on an outpatient basis, in and out in one day. Again, if you don't have to spend a night in the hospital, don't do it. Remember, any stay in a hospital entails money *and* potential exposure to unwanted illness.

<u>68.</u>

Go to the hospital that does the largest number of the procedure that you need.

Studies have shown that you are less likely to suffer complications or die if you have your surgery or other invasive procedure done at a hospital that performs a large number (some experts recommend at least 200 per year) of such procedures. You save yourself a lot of money and untold amounts of suffering if you do what you can to assure the best outcome from the start. After all, you pay the price in more than dollars for their mistakes or inadequacies.

<u>69.</u>

Avoid for-profit hospitals.

Along with the family farm, the independent community hospital is fast becoming a lone ranger. Hand in hand with the burgeoning for-profit hospital business has come a rise and monumental growth in corporate chain ownership. Today the top three for-profit medical corporations – Hospital Corporation of America, Humana, and American Medical International – either own or manage nearly 87,000 beds in 530 hospitals nationwide. Current estimates are that for-profit hospitals tend to be more expensive – as much as 23 percent more expensive. Recently, a particular for-profit hospital chain was found to have marked up supplies anywhere from a few hundred percent to 4,000 percent. Such economics may explain why a $3 pill costs up to $29 in one of these for-profit facilities. And who pays for this markup? You, your employer, and your insurance company all pay for these outrageous charges.

The savvy medical consumer's strategy is this: Before your doctor arranges for you to be admitted to a certain hospital (assuming, of course, that your condition does not require emergency care), find out who owns it and how that ownership might affect your care and its cost. Call the hospital and ask for the hospital administrator's office. Ask the administrator who owns the hospital. Ask if it is nonprofit, owned by a religious

order, or part of a large conglomerate that owns many more
facilities around the country. Know the setup before you become
a patient.

70.
Check room rates in advance.

There are differences in room rates from hospital to hospital. The
basic charge for a hospital room may vary from $250 to $500 a
day depending upon the type of hospital and region of the
country. The cost of ancillary services (lab, supplies, nursing,
etc.) can easily add an extra $500 a day. If you have an insurance
plan that pays only up to a certain amount, say $350 a day,
you've got to shop around for an affordable room.

71.
Refuse to pay a hospital admitting fee or hospital release (or discharge) fee to your doctor.

These fees, which are commonly charged by doctors for admitting
and discharging you from the hospital, are unjustifiable on the
basis of services rendered to you, the patient. Find out whether
your doctor customarily charges such fees and discuss your
objections prior to your admission to the hospital.

72.
Negotiate a discounted fee with your doctor in exchange for allowing services of a resident.

If you have no objection to having your surgery or other
procedures performed by a resident physician, then make that
clear to your doctor. Just remember that is how residents learn.
But make sure that you do not pay for more than you get.

73.
Avoid cesarean-section deliveries.

A recent study showed that more cesarean sections are performed at night and on weekends– partly because doctors want to get the delivery over with quickly and therefore are less willing to wait through a long labor.

Cesarean-section deliveries are major surgery. They are not only much more expensive than vaginal deliveries, but they also expose both mother and baby to additional risks. Further, studies show that only one out of four women who had a previous cesarean-section delivery need have another one for the birth of subsequent children. The adage of "Once a cesarean, always a cesarean" is just not true. Indeed, the American College of Obstetricians and Gynecologists issued strong guidelines some years back stating that repeat cesarean deliveries should no longer be routine.

The best way to avoid a cesarean-section delivery is to be as knowledgeable as you can about the birth process so that you will be better able to ask the right questions and evaluate your doctor's recommendations. Not all cesareans are avoidable, but a good many are–and with information on whys, wherefores, and options you can avoid being one of those.

74.
Use a nurse-midwife or family practitioner as your birth attendant and consider alternative birth settings.

At the outset let us say that, clearly, where birth attendants and settings are concerned, different strokes for different folks. The savvy–and pregnant–medical consumer realizes that the type of childbirth experience she has depends very much on who she finds to deliver her baby and where she decides to have it.

There are two reasons you save money by choosing a practitioner other than an obstetrician as your birth attendant: Other birth attendants usually charge less in basic delivery fees, and they generally will not recommend a costly cesarean section or other expensive (and potentially dangerous), high-technology interventions unless they are absolutely necessary. For more information on nurse-midwife services, contact:

American College of Nurse-Midwives
1522 K Street, N.W., Suite 1000
Washington, DC 20005
202-289-0171

Developed by midwives believing it to be the best alternative to both hospital and home deliveries, the birth center ideally offers a home*like* environment, a relaxed, flexible atmosphere, and very little intervention in the birth process. Birth centers are designed to provide maternity care to women judged to be at low risk of obstetric complications, and this approach enjoys a loyal following of doctors, midwives, childbirth educators, and consumers who champion the low complication and cesarean-section rates, safety, consumer satisfaction, and cost savings that many birth centers offer. A 1989 survey showed that, for normal birth, birth centers offer a 35 to 47 percent cost savings over hospitals, depending on the length of stay. For more information, contact:

National Association of Childbearing Centers
3123 Gottschall Road
Perkiomenville, PA 18074
215-234-8068

There is also growing interest in home births, and if your insurance plan will cover such services it's worthwhile to investigate your options. For more information, contact:

National Association of Parents and Professionals for
    Safe Alternatives in Childbirth
Route 1, Box 646
Marble Hill, MO 63764
314-238-2010

75.

Become acquainted with the hospital's birthing policies and routine services before choosing to deliver there.

From a cost perspective, you should be looking for hospital policies that encourage "rooming-in" (keeping the baby in the room with you) and early discharge (generally after 24 hours rather than three days). Often hospitals charge for routine birth services – such as enemas, IVs, and use of the delivery room – that not every woman has. Scrutinize the bill and don't pay for any service you didn't receive. (And don't permit your insurance company to either.) By the way, the average charge for a hospital-based birth is $4,300 ($7,200 for a cesarean section).

76.

Do not routinely circumcise your male babies.

Circumcision is an operative procedure for which hospitals charge around $75. It is recognized to be unnecessary for health reasons; consequently, more and more health insurance companies are refusing to pay for this procedure. For more information, contact:

> National Organization of Circumcision Information
>   Resource Centers
> P. O. Box 2512
> San Anselmo, CA 94979-2512

77.

Demand itemized bills.

Ongoing studies by national hospital bill auditing firms consistently show that upwards of 90 percent of all hospital bills contain errors – miscalculations that are seldom in your, the consumer's, favor. In fact, the situation has gotten so out of hand that businesses are now offering "bounties" to employees who can spot the inaccuracies in their bills. The reward is a split of the money recovered from the hospital.

The problem here is that you can spot these errors only if you receive an itemized bill, which in most cases will not be given to you unless you ask for it. Scrutinize the bill closely, looking for any supplies, services, procedures, tests, or whatever that you did not receive.

If your bill is going to be paid by your insurer, be sure to inform your insurer directly, and in writing, of any inaccuracies in the bill. Everyone saves money by making sure that insurers do not overpay hospitals.

HOSPITAL BILLING ERRORS: WHAT TO LOOK FOR

American Claims Evaluation, Inc., another firm in the business of auditing hospital bills, recommends that you ask yourself the following questions to help identify possible errors on a bill. Clearly, these do not cover every possible misbilling, but they are a good start:

1. Was I billed for the right kind of room (semiprivate, private, etc.)?
2. Was I billed for the correct number of days I occupied the hospital room?
3. Was I billed correctly for any time spent in specialized units (intensive care unit, coronary care unit, etc.)?
4. If I left before "checkout time," was I billed for an extra day even though I'd already gone?
5. Was I billed only for those X rays and tests that I actually received?
6. If I had preadmission testing, did the hospital bill me for the "standard admission test battery" even though I never had it?
7. Was I charged only for supplies, medications, therapy, dressings, injections, etc., that I received? Were the quantities correct?
8. Were medications that my doctor prescribed billed over the entire stay even though I took them only once or twice?
9. Were drugs prescribed for me to take home actually received?
10. Was I billed for bedpans, humidifiers, admission kits, thermometers, etc., that I never received and/or was not allowed to take home?

78.
Keep a diary to compare with the hospital bill.

Document all medications, tests, and procedures, and compare your list with the itemized hospital bill. Make sure that individual items match those you actually received, and that you are not billed for more items than you received. Again, if you didn't use or undergo it, don't pay for it. You'll find a complete hospital diary in the back of the People's Medical Society book *Take This Book To The Hospital With You* (New York: Pantheon, 1991), along with a hospital evaluation form that should be sent to the People's Medical Society.

79.
Make sure you get what you pay for.

Many hospitals are teaching hospitals, which means they have a staff of medical interns and residents who work with "attending" physicians (such as your doctor). Unfortunately, this means that although you are paying full fees to your doctor, he may be doing very little of the work. You should specify, in writing, that any surgery or invasive procedure be done by the person you are paying for the service. If you are paying for a fully-trained physician, that is who you should get.

80.
Refuse to be seen by any doctor you don't know.

If any doctor you do not know enters your hospital room to see you, you can be sure you will receive a bill for his "services" (often nothing more than a quick glance into your room) unless you immediately make it clear that you do not want those services. Find out who these doctors are and why they are there, and make sure you or your insurer does not pay later for the services.

81.
Have a friend or relative with you to act as advocate.

As a hospital patient, it is very difficult to be an assertive consumer. Always bring along a friend or family member to act as an advocate, whose most important task will be to make sure you do not agree to anything without fully understanding it. In many cases, these personal advocates may have to stay with you 24 hours a day.

Many hospitals have on staff a so-called patient advocate, who supposedly can help you resolve minor problems. While we can't vouch for the effectiveness of every patient advocate, it's a good idea to at least become acquainted with this person. Let this person know that you're an informed consumer and won't hesitate to call upon him if a situation should arise. And don't forget to bring to the hospital your copy of *Take This Book To The Hospital With You,* the People's Medical Society's guide to surviving your hospital stay.

82.
Die at home.

Over 50 percent of medical costs are incurred in the last five days of life. Of course, the decision about where to die is very personal and one that many never get the opportunity to make. But it is a valid consideration – for many reasons, including cost – and should be given serious thought.

83.
Make a living will.

A living will is a legal document that is used to inform family and medical personnel of your wishes concerning medical care, should you be unable to personally make those wishes known. These documents are most often used to limit the types of medical care you wish to receive if you are known to be in a terminal stage of illness. For instance, a living will may proscribe the use of an artificial life-sustaining treatment, such as an automatic ventilator.

As of 1992 every hospital is required by law to ask you if you have a living will or any other type of directive that can be followed if the issue should arise. The law does not require you to have such directives nor does it mean you must make one up. It merely requires hospitals to ask.

There are many reasons, in addition to the cost considerations, to choose to have a living will. No matter what your reasons, it is a good idea to discuss your living will with both your family and your doctor. And prepare your family to fight for your right to the choices expressed in the living will should you personally be unable to do so.

If you do have a living will, make sure you give a copy to your family doctor and any other physician you regularly use. If you are brought to a hospital unconscious or with no family member present, contact may be made with one of these doctors, who can then pass along your instructions.

To obtain more information on living wills and durable power of attorney for health care – the latter, another form of advance directive – contact:

> Choice in Dying, Inc.
> 250 West 57th Street
> New York, NY 10107
> 212-246-6973

84.
Bring your own food.

Hospital meals are expensive (and, frankly, not always edible), partly because of the costs of hiring clinical dietitians who order menus based upon patients' nutritional needs. But if you are permitted to eat a normal diet, you will not need any special food and can save a lot of money – and keep your taste buds happy in the process – by providing your own food. (Skeptics of hospital food – and there are many, including probably most people who have ever eaten such food – maintain that you won't miss much either.) This strategy may also be necessary if you are on a restricted, such as vegetarian or kosher, diet. Remember, though, that providing three meals per day is hospital routine. So make it explicit that you do not want the meals and will not pay for them.

85.
Bring your own drugs.

This is a savvy (and easy) money-saving technique. Bring to the hospital an adequate supply of any medications you take (making sure beforehand, of course, that your doctor is aware of your usual medication regimen and has documented such in your hospital record). Medicate yourself at the appropriate times. It is also a good idea to take along some basic analgesics such as aspirin or acetaminophen, if you use them. Hospitals charge a lot ($3 for two aspirin tablets, in some cases) for medications.

If you are unable to medicate yourself, ask a family member to help. Have your doctor inform the nurses of such an arrangement.

86.
Bring your own vitamins to the hospital.

Hospitals do not ordinarily supply vitamin or mineral supplements—and if they did, you can be sure it would be at an exorbitant price. So if you customarily follow a vitamin and mineral supplementation regimen, bring them with you. And make sure the doctor marks on your chart that you are to be given your own vitamins, or that supplements are to stay in your possession so you can take them yourself.

87.
Avoid weekend admission.

Don't allow yourself to be admitted on a nonemergency basis on a Friday afternoon or evening. You will just languish, expensively and in no particular comfort, until Monday. Most of the labs that would be performing your diagnostic workups don't do those things on weekends. Weekend admission equals one to two days extra in the hospital, at your expense. Only basic care is performed on the weekend. Wait until Monday; better yet, Tuesday, some experts say. By Tuesday the hospital is back in gear after the weekend and the end-of-the-week blahs haven't hit yet.

88.
Complain if you are being disturbed.

Hospital personnel are accustomed to dealing with uncomplaining, often drugged patients. If your room is noisy at night or your sleep is disturbed, complain. A *British Medical Journal* report some years back cited more than 20 studies that responded resoundingly yes to the question "Is sound, prolonged sleep essential for optimal healing?" The savvy medical consumer will make sure that adequate rest periods of uninterrupted sleep are part of the care plan.

CHAPTER 4

Laboratories

Over- and unnecessary testing and errors in test results are problems you've got to be on the lookout for. They can do irreparable harm to your pocketbook—*and your health*, if you undergo a dangerous invasive procedure as a result of a faulty test result. A former editor of the American Medical Association's own journal has estimated that more than half of the tens of millions of medical tests performed yearly "do not really contribute to a patient's diagnosis or therapy." And the Centers for Disease Control have found that as much as 50 percent of simple blood and urine chemistry tests done in the top 10 percent of the laboratories in the U.S. are inaccurate. All lab test results can be expected to be incorrect a certain percentage of the time, so even the healthiest person will have an abnormal test result from time to time.

There's also the issue of defensive medicine. If the term is new to you, it is doctor-speak meaning "I gotta do the test because if I don't the litigious patient might later sue me if something goes wrong." Physicians are subjecting unsuspecting (and usually litigiously low-risk) customers to a battery of worthless pokes and probes that would send Hippocrates, if he were alive today, back to his famed Oath to add a new canon (after "First, do no harm"), which would state "Second, do no unnecessary test."

What can you do? Ensure that you have tests only when necessary and retest when appropriate. Here's how you do it:

89.

Avoid hospital laboratories and laboratories and imaging centers owned by doctors.

Hospital labs are no more reliable than independent laboratories, and they are usually considerably more expensive because the hospital overhead (cost of building, equipment, utilities) is higher.

Also, don't use a laboratory or imaging center that is owned by the physician making the referral. It just stands to reason. No judge should preside over a case in which she has a personal, vested interest. So why then let physicians refer patients to X-ray labs, specialty clinics, private hospitals, kidney dialysis units, and physical therapy practices that these same physicians either own or have a financial interest in?

In medicine it's called referral for profit, although more hard-nosed critics have labeled it a kickback scheme. The latest evidence is that doctors who have a financial interest in laboratories order four times the number of diagnostic tests as physicians with no financial investment. And a General Accounting Office study found that physician-owners of Maryland labs or imaging centers ordered, on average, 14 percent more expensive lab tests and 82 percent more expensive imaging tests than nonowner doctors.

How prevalent are these joint ventures, these investments in health care facilities by physicians in positions to refer patients for tests or services? An important Florida study, released in August 1991, found that at least 40 percent of the doctors practicing in that state have invested in joint ventures to which they can refer patients. So be on guard against the doctor more interested in protecting his investment than in healing the sick.

90.

Don't let the laboratory run more tests than you need.

You will notice that lab forms, particularly for blood and urine tests, list a number of different tests on one slip. Make sure that you and your doctor clearly indicate the specific tests that you need. Otherwise, the lab may run all the tests on the lab slip and you will be charged for them.

Routine presurgical lab tests are another problem area. They account for $30 billion a year in business, yet researchers have found that nearly half the time the tests duplicate those that patients had within the previous year. The findings indicate that normal results taken up to four months prior to surgery can be substituted safely for preoperative screening tests.

91.

If your doctor recommends an invasive procedure as the result of a laboratory test, request a retest before agreeing to the procedure.

Because of the large numbers of errors made in laboratory tests, it makes sense both financially and for the sake of your health to pay the small fee for another lab test. Erroneous lab results can expose you to expensive, dangerous, and potentially life-threatening invasive procedures. If your insurance plan requires approval for any retesting, just remind the powers-that-be that a $25 or $35 retest can save thousands in future expenses, not to mention out-of-pocket costs that are your responsibility.

92.

Investigate the use of home tests rather than laboratory tests.

Consumers are doing more to keep the doctor away, or at bay, than just eating an apple a day. Sales of do-it-yourself medical tests a few years ago topped the $500-million-a-year mark, and the best predictions have sales climbing to $1.4 billion in 1992. Sold in drugstores, in supermarkets, and through catalogs, home tests make it possible for you to take your own blood pressure, check yourself for a urinary tract infection, determine whether you're pregnant, screen yourself for certain cancers, monitor your blood sugar levels, and even predict when you're ovulating. Home testing offers a low-cost, convenient alternative to the doctor's office or lab, at least in the early stages of diagnosis.

But aside from the cost-containment angle, such testing is a good idea because it enables the consumer to involve herself in self-care and in aspects of health care once exclusively the doctor's domain. Do-it-yourself tests, however, are not without potential problems—accuracy, for one, and the situation in which your doctor just repeats the test you took at home. Most experts agree that the objective of home medical tests is for you to *work together* with your health professional to ensure the best health for yourself. Your pharmacist is a good source of information on home medical tests and can tell you what is presently available.

Remember too that not all home testing requires a kit. According to the American Cancer Society, every woman over 20 should examine her breasts monthly. Also, the most common type of cancer in humans, skin cancer, is largely curable if caught early, and you don't need a kit to check your skin for moles and suspicious and rapid changes in them.

93.
Take advantage of free testing programs at community health fairs.

Usually sponsored by hospitals and featuring a lot of giveaways along the lines of refrigerator magnets and such, health fairs offer simple screening tests: blood pressure, cholesterol, and tuberculosis screening; blood typing; vision testing, and on and on. Since these screenings are usually free, the greatest cost advantage is that you avoid having to pay for a doctor's visit unless one of the test results indicates that you need a doctor's care.

Most health fairs are set up for the purpose of getting the consumer to use (translate: buy) the services of the participating facilities or physicians. In the words of a top medical marketer, writing in *Medical Economics*, "Doctors looking for an inexpensive way to attract more patients frequently sign up with health fairs . . . just the kind of low-key marketing that many physicians like best." In other words, keep a cautious attitude, and make sure the fair promoters are providing a community service—not just an opportunity for doctors and hospitals to make a quick buck (or several hundred and more) off you.

CHAPTER 5

Insurance

Everyone hopes to stay healthy–but since there's a good chance you or a member of your family will get sick at some point, it's smart to know how to shop for the best health insurance for your money.

Most people carry health insurance, if they can afford it, or have it provided as a benefit of employment. Lately, though, you've probably noticed that your coverage is not as extensive as it once was and you're paying more in out-of-pocket expenses for deductibles and copayments. Some employers, who once provided cost-free health insurance, now require employees to make premium contributions.

For some time now, business interests have contended that their cost to provide health insurance has been increasing at a rate of 14 percent or more per year, which they say they can no longer tolerate. As a result, some companies have purchased health insurance plans that pay fewer benefits. This leaves you, the employee, facing larger and larger out-of-pocket expenses. The goal then is to maximize your health insurance benefits and reduce your out-of-pocket expense as much as possible. Here's how:

94.
Don't duplicate coverage.

Chances are you will not be permitted to collect full benefits from both policies. The insurance companies invoke a policy they call coordination of benefits, which means they compare notes to determine who owes what. They split the bill, or at least the portion that is their responsibility, and you still must pick up any copayment or deductible. In essence then, the premium for the second policy is down the drain.

95.
Don't buy disease-specific or accident insurance.

Disease-specific insurance usually covers one disease—for example, cancer or heart disease—and not only pays limited benefits but may duplicate what you already have or are about to purchase. Very limited in coverage (and for this reason not the best insurance for your money), accident insurance excludes illness but does cover medical expenses resulting from an accident. And most insurers will not allow you to collect from more than one policy for a single injury.

96.
Shop carefully for long-term-care insurance.

This insurance is also known as nursing home insurance. The most important point to ask is whether benefits are paid for any level of care: skilled, intermediate, or custodial. It's important to make sure the policy you buy pays for all three levels. Early on, long-term-care insurance paid benefits only for skilled nursing care, but today policies usually cover the full range of services available. The benefits are paid when such services are deemed medically necessary.

97.
Take advantage of the "free look" period.

After you have signed the application and paid the premium, your state may permit you to review the policy for a certain number of days—most allow 10 to 15 days—before you decide whether or not to keep it. If you are not satisfied and decide not to keep the policy, return it to the company within the time allotted and request a full refund of any premium. Call your state insurance department if you have any questions about your policy or about your state's "free look" regulation.

98.
Ask if your employer pays bounty for erroneous medical bills.

The first question a savvy medical consumer asks is "How good are my chances of finding errors?" Equifax Services, an Atlanta firm that audits around 40,000 hospital bills annually for insurers, found in one audit of selected bills that more than 97 percent of hospital bills contain errors. When the *Philadelphia Daily News* took a look at billing—again, hospital bills, in particular—in that city, it found case after case of erroneous charges. In one case, a man had his $25,185 bill for a two-week hospital stay reduced by more than $2,000 after an auditor discovered overcharges.

Many companies will pay a reward, or "bounty," to an employee who finds inaccuracies in her hospital bill that result in savings to the company. And, as you can imagine, it shouldn't be too difficult to find an error; national studies indicate that upwards of 90 percent of all hospital bills contain errors—usually in the hospital's favor. Your vigilance not only helps reduce your copayment, but your employer also benefits from the overall reduction in health insurance costs.

Don't be surprised if your insurer is not overly enthusiastic when you call to report a hospital's or doctor's overcharge. Not every company pays a reward—or even pays attention—to such diligence on your part. Insurance companies often find it easier to pay erroneous claims rather than go to the trouble of auditing the bill and possibly demanding a refund. But you and everyone else pay for overcharges, so be persistent. Be prepared to fight with your insurer over an error in your bill.

99.

Get preapproval to make sure services are covered.

Many insurance companies encourage preapproval for any procedure your doctor recommends. This just means that you submit a request to your insurance company, who will then either approve or disapprove coverage for the recommended procedure. The process of preapproval becomes even more important when there are penalties attached to bypassing the system. You may opt to have a procedure or treatment done without approval only to learn that your coverage has been reduced by half. Remember, no matter how insistent your doctor is, always check with your insurance carrier prior to any service.

100.

Pay premiums annually if you can afford to.

You may be able to receive a discount on your premium if you can pay yearly in one lump sum, or even on a semiannual basis. If you don't have an insurance plan where you work, consider asking your employer to pick up part of the premium. This way you can make the yearly premium payment and obtain a small benefit from your employment. It also saves your employer the full cost of starting a medical benefits plan.

101.

Check out local HMOs and PPOs—they may be cheaper than health insurance and offer better benefits.

Health maintenance organizations (HMOs) and preferred provider organizations (PPOs) are forms of health insurance policies as well as providers. Managed-care plans, as they are often called, are sometimes referred to as alternative delivery systems, which simply means alternatives to the traditional fee-for-service system. For the savvy medical consumer, the time to learn the rudiments of managed-care plans is *now*—as the popularity of these plans increases every year and more employers drop traditional insurance entirely and offer managed-care plans or nothing.

Health maintenance organizations come in a variety of forms, but with some elements in common:

► HMO members (usually called subscribers) receive comprehensive medical care for a fixed (or prepaid, meaning paid before you receive the services) monthly premium.

► The services are provided by an organized group of medical professionals who receive a fixed monthly payment per subscriber, regardless of the services rendered (or not rendered, whatever the case may be).

► Subscribers, for the most part, are limited to those physicians, hospitals, and other medical providers approved by the HMO.

A preferred provider organization, or PPO, is a group of physicians and hospitals that contract with insurance companies, unions, or employers to provide health care at negotiated fees. In return, the "preferred" group is guaranteed a volume of patients.

You need to find out when the HMOs in your area have open enrollment periods, and whether or not you meet the enrollment criteria. Also speak to your employer about offering an HMO as an option to traditional health insurance – if your company does not already. If your company offers a PPO, be aware that by joining it you will be severely limited in the providers you may use.

Consider what it would mean to you to change doctors or use a hospital that is not your favorite, should these be limitations set by the HMO or PPO. In either case, compare rates and coverage. HMOs and PPOs may (or may not) be cheaper.

102.
Use only providers who accept your insurance plan.

Some health insurers have arrangements with certain doctors and hospitals – called "participating" providers. Your policy will reimburse at a higher level if you use a participating provider.

103.

See if you're eligible for group insurance through organizations or associations to which you belong.

If you are unemployed or otherwise without an employer-subsidized health insurance policy, you may be able to obtain a less expensive group policy through organizations or associations to which you belong–and you may not have to look any further than your mailbox. Many fraternal, alumni, and civic associations have health insurance plans for sale. While many of these offerings are indemnity plans–i.e., they pay a fixed amount per day in the hospital or per service–in a pinch they can cover at least some of your expenses.

Some states are now offering low-cost insurance for disabled and/or handicapped persons who are unable to obtain private insurance. Contact your state insurance department or department of welfare to see if it is available where you live and if you are eligible.

104.

Donate blood—join a blood bank.

By committing yourself to the donation of a specified amount of blood per year, you can receive insurance coverage for blood supplies for yourself and possibly for your family as well.

105.

Join an ambulance service.

Just as with a blood bank, private and voluntary ambulance services will often offer a specified amount of service for a yearly donation.

106.
Check all employer-sponsored health insurance plan options carefully.

A happy scenario is one where your employer, as many larger companies are doing, offers a wide range of policies and options at varying costs. Many workers are offered a "cafeteria package" of benefits and must choose from an assortment of possibilities. Unfortunately, too many people decide by the toss of a coin—an uninformed and hardly savvy decision-making tactic. To get the best value for your money, carefully compare all the policies with *your needs* in mind. Do not settle for less coverage than you need. Your premium for more coverage may not be much higher.

107.
Pay premiums on time.

An insurance company can cancel your policy if you fail to pay the premiums or continually pay the premiums late. Be sure to keep on top of any necessary employee deductions if yours is an employer-sponsored policy.

108.
Know what your state insurance department can do for you in the way of consumer protection.

Your state insurance department plays an important role in regulating insurance companies. Beyond licensing insurance companies and agents, approving policies that are sold, and mandating minimum benefits for policies—the department has the power to conduct investigations, take testimony, hold hearings, and render verdicts. As such, your state insurance department may also be able to help you if you have a problem with an insurance company or agent. Any formal complaint you file with the department will be investigated and, if possible, resolved.

HOW TO FILE A COMPLAINT
WITH YOUR STATE INSURANCE DEPARTMENT

Your complaint should be in writing and contain the following information:

► Your name, address, and telephone number.

► The name, address, and telephone number of your insurance company.

► The identification number of your policy.

► The type of policy.

► The nature of your complaint: the premium, the coverage, a claim, or the actions of your agent.

Make sure you keep copies of everything you send to the department. You must be willing to follow through on your complaint and appear at any hearings if so directed. If the law and the facts are on your side, the insurance department can usually help resolve the problem.

CHAPTER 6

Nursing Home and Home Health Care

The term "nursing home" is actually a very general name for several different types of medical care facilities. It has the connotation of being a "last stop" for the elderly, but it can actually be a place for people of all ages to convalesce following an accident or serious illness, or a temporary placement for an older person while the family shops around and lines up alternative modes of care. A common classification for nursing homes is the level of care they provide:

▶ *Skilled nursing.* Care is delivered by registered and licensed practical nurses on the orders of an attending physician. The person who requires skilled nursing is often bedridden and not able to help himself or herself.

▶ *Intermediate care.* The intermediate care facility provides less intensive care than the skilled facility and usually costs less; the care there stresses rehabilitation therapy to enable the resident to go home or at least regain or retain as many functions of daily living as possible. Care is delivered by registered and licensed practical nurses and an array of therapists.

▶ *Sheltered, or custodial, care.* This level of care is nonmedical in that residents do not require constant attention from nurses or aides, but do need help with such routine activities as getting out of bed, walking, eating, and bathing.

One in every five people can expect to need extended nursing care at some time in their lives. To make matters worse, very few basic health insurance policies cover nursing home care for more than a few days or weeks. Even Medicare, the federal health insurance plan for senior citizens, does not cover what we think of as long-term care. Medicare covers a limited number of days of skilled nursing facility care only, and is primarily intended to permit recovery outside of a hospital. So if you or a member of your family needs such care, you must know how to get quality care without paying more than necessary.

What follows are ways for the savvy medical consumer to get the best value in extended nursing care. Knowing all of your options is the key.

109.

Check the yellow pages for the visiting nurse association and other agencies that provide home health care.

The first thing to know is that nursing home placement is not, and should not be, the sole solution to the plight of an older person who is debilitated by ill health and who has increasing difficulty taking care of himself or herself. Nothing mandates nursing home placement if there is someone available to administer the needed care in the home or to coordinate delivery of alternative services. Visiting nurse associations (VNAs) are the oldest home health care agencies in most communities; however, they aren't the only agencies that provide home health services. Hospitals, not-for-profit community organizations, and for-profit agencies are also in the home care business. VNAs provide referrals to other community services when appropriate.

Familiarize yourself with the various levels of care available in your community. Full-service agencies, such as the VNA and certified home health agencies, offer everything from skilled nursing care to homemaker services. If you're responsible for the full cost of the services, don't contract for more care than you need. Another important point to consider is whether or not the agency is certified. This could become rather important if your health insurance plan will cover only services from a certified agency. These groups can provide you with information on certified home care agencies:

National League for Nursing
350 Hudson Street
New York, NY 10014
212-989-9393

Joint Commission on the Accreditation of
    Healthcare Organizations
One Renaissance Boulevard
Oakbrook, IL 60181
708-916-5600

National HomeCaring Council
519 C Street, N.E.
Washington, DC 20002
202-547-6586

For information on home health services, contact:

Foundation for Hospice and Home Care
519 C Street, N.E.
Washington, DC 20002
202-547-6586

National Association for Home Care
519 C Street, N.E.
Washington, DC 20002
202-547-7424

110.
Use adult day care.

An adult day care center lets an elderly person enjoy a full range
of activities–including arts and crafts, games, and just plain old
conversation–on a daily basis in a supervised setting. Communities nationwide are establishing such facilities, which provide a
degree of supervision and appropriate activities for elderly persons
with minor physical disabilities but do not provide nursing care.

It is well established that elderly people remain healthier if
they are able to continue to live in their own homes–and it's
usually cheaper, too. Adult day care can often make the
difference between being able to remain at home and needing
institutionalization.

111.

Use home health care.

Home health agencies can provide services ranging from help with cooking and cleaning to full nursing care at home. For the elderly person with minor disabilities, a person to cook or clean is often all the support that's needed. A home health agency can help you evaluate the help that you need. But don't purchase any more care than necessary.

Bear in mind too that home health care is not just for the elderly on Medicare. Many people under age 65, who are not yet legally disabled—and who therefore would not normally qualify for Medicare—but who require rehabilitative or chronic care, are eligible to use home care programs. Home health services offer an opportunity for early discharge from a hospital or a skilled nursing facility, and in fact such specialized or rehabilitation services often meet a person's long-term needs more efficiently than acute care hospital settings.

If you are eligible for Medicare, know the limits of coverage of home health care. If you are not on Medicare, find out what your insurance plan pays and what eligibility requirements you must meet. Generally, a doctor must arrange for such services as part-time home nursing care, occupational therapy, speech therapy, and special meals and other nutritional services to be furnished in your home.

112.

If you need nursing home care, purchase the lowest level necessary.

Of the three levels of nursing home care—skilled, intermediate, and custodial—skilled care is the most expensive because care is provided by registered and licensed practical nurses on the orders of an attending physician. Remember, skilled care is the only level of care that Medicare will reimburse for, and then only a very limited amount of coverage is provided.

For information on nursing home care, contact:

American Health Care Association
1201 L Street, N.W.
Washington, DC 20005
202-842-4444

American Association of Homes for the Aging
901 E Street, N.W., Suite 500
Washington, DC 20004
202-783-2242

National Consumers League
815 15th Street, N.W., Suite 928
Washington, DC 20005
202-639-8140

QUICK CHECKLIST OF QUESTIONS FOR NURSING HOME ADMINISTRATORS

Even before you spend your time going around to various nursing homes, touring them, and interviewing administrators, you should conduct phone interviews to establish a base of information on which to build. Find out:

1. What level of care is offered?
2. Are there special restrictions on the types of patients accepted?
3. How many beds (for the type of care you need) does the home provide?
4. Is there a waiting list, and if so, approximately how long is it?
5. What type of license or accreditation does the home have?
6. Does the home accept Medicare and Medicaid?
7. Is there an initial deposit required, and, if so, how much is it?
8. What are the monthly room charges?
9. Are additional monthly services provided? What are their charges?

113.

Use Meals on Wheels and/or other programs that are alternatives to institutionalization.

An excellent program designed to provide hot, nutritious meals to homebound older people, Meals on Wheels is usually operated by a social service agency or community group. The service delivers one hot meal a day directly to the person's residence, and the price of such a service is nominal, often based on ability to pay.

As with a number of other programs for those people who do not require constant supervision or that much nursing care, Meals on Wheels may actually delay a person's need for a nursing home for many years. The savvy medical consumer will explore the other programs as well: *homemaker services*, for people who require some assistance in the preparation of meals or with housework; *home sharing*, an arrangement in which a resident manager and a few older people share housing and share expenses; *telephone reassurance*, a formal or informal system to take away the risk of total isolation for the elderly person living alone; *shopping services*, which entail having groceries and other needed items delivered; *special transportation services*, consisting of vehicles equipped to handle wheelchairs and other devices, for people with limited mobility; and *special health aids or devices*, such as walkers, mechanical feeding devices, geriatric chairs, and artificial limbs, which can facilitate personal independence or make it more feasible for a family member to assist. Contact your local, county, or state welfare or human services agencies for availability of or more information about these programs.

114.

Use a hospice.

Hospices are for people who are terminally ill, and their mission is to inspirit death with dignity and allow the family close contact with the patient, free from the intrusive high technology of the hospital. Less expensive than a hospital because they do not use life-sustaining technologies, a hospice provides basic medical care, counseling for the patient and family, and prescribed pain relievers. Most hospices will care for patients for whom a doctor's prognosis indicates that they have fewer than six months to live. Some hospices come to a person's home and provide services, while others actually operate a facility where the patient resides. For information on hospice care, contact:

> Children's Hospice International
> 901 N. Washington Street, Suite 700
> Alexandria, VA 22314
> 800-242-4453

> Hospice Education Institute
> 5 Essex Square, Suite 3-B
> Essex, CT 06426
> 800-331-1620

> National Hospice Organization
> 1901 North Moore Street, Suite 901
> Alexandria, VA 22209
> 800-658-8898

115.
Investigate life care communities.

A relatively new concept, these communities provide residential care in an apartment-like setting, along with skilled and intermediate nursing care. As residents require nursing care, they are transferred to the nursing home section of the community, and once they recover return to their apartments. The life care community covers all costs of hospitalization, so, as you can imagine, the services do not come cheap. This option often requires a substantial, nonrefundable down payment as well as monthly fees. A good source of information on life care communities is available from:

> American Association of Homes for the Aging
> 901 E Street, N.W., Suite 500
> Washington, DC 20004
> 202-783-2242

116.

Prepare for the financial costs of nursing home care.

Nursing home care is expensive, costing you anywhere from $20,000 to $35,000 per year, depending on the level of care. Many insurance companies are now offering long-term-care insurance–specifically designed to cover nursing home care. If you're going to purchase such a policy, a good rule of thumb is to select a policy that pays at least $60 per day, for a period of at least four years. Look for a policy that will keep up with inflation. A present benefit of $60 a day could easily dwindle to a future value of only $20 due to inflation. To obtain a list of insurance companies offering long-term-care policies, contact:

Health Insurance Association of America
P. O. Box 41455
Washington, DC 20018

Also look into your eligibility for Medicaid. Medicaid is the government health insurance program that will pay for nursing home care when most of a person's assets have been depleted. The fact is that most people in nursing homes for any length of time usually end up using the Medicaid program.

CHAPTER 7

Medical Equipment

Durable medical equipment such as hospital beds and wheel-chairs can be extremely valuable tools in caring for an ill person at home—*and* can save you money in the process. Anything that enables a sick person to remain at home rather than in an institution makes dollars and sense.

Now the bad news. According to recent government reports, some unethical medical equipment companies have targeted Medicare beneficiaries as easy marks for purchasing medical equipment. The scam usually starts with a letter or telephone call to beneficiaries telling them that they are eligible for a particular piece of medical equipment and that Medicare will pay for it. The problem here is that the equipment may or may not be needed, and if it isn't medically necessary Medicare will not pay for it. And guess who gets stuck with the bill?

If you know what to look for and what to do, you can save money on durable medical equipment. Here are our suggestions:

117.
Borrow medical equipment whenever possible.

Most home health aids can be borrowed from various community organizations. Ask your local home health organization or visiting nurse association. If no such services are available in your area, you may be able to rent the required equipment from a local pharmacy. But before renting, check to see if your insurance policy will cover its purchase. Also shop around; rental prices for equipment vary from dealer to dealer. If you need the equipment for a long period of time, you will probably have to purchase it.

118.
Save by owning medical self-care equipment.

Simple self-care equipment such as thermometers, blood pressure cuffs, stethoscopes, and otoscopes are helpful devices, especially when it comes to making informed choices concerning your need for doctor's help. Many are available from discount mail-order companies. Check out a number of suppliers to find a high quality item at a reasonable price.

119.
Check out the equipment's reliability before purchasing.

Every piece of equipment you purchase should come with literature that describes its reliability within a certain range. For instance, thermometers may be reliable within a range of one degree Fahrenheit. Some equipment will be more reliable than others. The equipment's accompanying literature should also describe the period of time the equipment can be expected to maintain this degree of reliability without servicing.

120.
Find out where servicing is available.

Equipment such as blood pressure cuffs must be periodically serviced to maintain reliability. Make sure that you know how, where, and how often a piece of equipment must be serviced before you purchase it. In fact, it makes sense to purchase only equipment with a written warranty. Further, you will save money if the equipment you buy can be serviced locally.

121.

Check the supplier with the Better Business Bureau, and with Medicare if the equipment is for a Medicare beneficiary.

For many health items such as hearing aids, it is wise to see if your local Better Business Bureau has any complaints on file against the supplier from whom you are thinking of purchasing. If the equipment is prescribed for a Medicare beneficiary, determine if the supplier is a certified Medicare supplier. What this means is that the supplier will accept the Medicare-approved amount as payment in full and will bill the beneficiary only for the 20 percent copayment.

122.

Check for sales.

With health and medical equipment, just as with most other consumer items, suppliers often offer sales. Purchasing items on sale is always a good way to save money.

123.

Return any medical equipment that arrives unsolicited.

Some doctors and medical suppliers target Medicare beneficiaries with offers of so-called free equipment paid for by Medicare. In addition, some equipment manufacturers use well-known personalities to hawk various products ranging from special beds to power-assisted chairs. Be aware that Medicare will pay only for durable medical equipment that's ordered by your doctor, as long as it is medically necessary. The words "medically necessary" are the key here. Unless your doctor specifically orders equipment, do not respond to any mail order or telephone marketing schemes.

CHAPTER 8

Prevention

Preventive measures have the potential to save you more
money on health costs than anything else you do. Even more
important, prevention is health promotion, something every
savvy medical consumer should be doing more of. But the bad
news is that—as 58 cents out of every health care dollar go to
doctors and hospitals—only two cents go to health promotion
activities. That's all we spend to keep ourselves healthy.

However, you have many opportunities in daily living to get
your two cents' worth by doing things to improve your health.
Remember, the sooner you start, the healthier you will be.

124.
Learn stress-reduction techniques.

There are techniques—some simple, others requiring professional
help—that can help you lower your stress level. Strong evidence
exists that those under stress, or those who cope poorly with
stress, are less healthy than others. And at the very least that adds
up to a lot of extra dollars spent on medical care.

125.
Quit smoking.

Smoking increases a person's risk for a number of major diseases:
heart disease, stroke, and cancer. But beyond that, smokers are

just generally more prone to illness—and therefore lose more work time due to illness—than nonsmokers. If you are a smoker, consider also the increased risk at which you put your friends and family as they breathe in your exhaled smoke. Save money and your health by throwing away your cigarettes.

126.
Don't do anything to excess.

Old wisdom, but true today. Excessive eating, drinking, smoking, and even exercise can be harmful and expensive.

127.
Make your home injury-proof.

Inspect your home for safety. Check electrical cords, the condition of carpeting, the placement of furniture, and so on. Additions such as nonslip strips on bathtubs are inexpensive ways to ensure your safety and prevent the need for costly medical care.

128.
Maintain desirable weight.

This does not necessarily mean that you should weigh what those famous charts say you should weigh, but you will be healthier if you weigh what feels good for you. And you'll save money on health care as well.

129.
Wear seat belts.

Many new cars employ a passive-restraint system that automatically fastens your seat belt; however, you may still need to manually fasten the lap belt. Whatever the case, you're always safer when you use the safety equipment that is included with your car. Fifty thousand deaths a year, untold pain and suffering, and loss of income should be enough to convince anyone to use seat belts.

130.
Always properly restrain children in cars.

Remember—*you* are responsible for the safety of your children. It's a good idea to take along a car seat on airplanes and other forms of transportation, too. Injury prevention saves money and incalculable suffering.

131.
Avoid processed foods.

Processed foods usually contain more fat, more salt, and less fiber than unprocessed foods. They also contain preservatives and other chemicals. The healthier you are, the more money you will save on costly medical care—so pass the bran.

132.
Have microwave emissions checked.

Call the authorized repair service recommended in the literature accompanying your microwave. (Indeed, your manual should include a maintenance schedule.) A repair service should be able to do a quick, low-cost emission check. Microwave emissions are potentially harmful, so a few dollars for a check can save you medical costs in the future.

133.
Purchase basic medical tools for self-diagnosis.

You can save yourself time and expense by having basic medical tools such as a blood pressure cuff (sphygmomanometer), an otoscope (for looking in the ears), and a stethoscope. Used in combination with a good medical guide, you can avoid many unnecessary visits to the doctor.

134.
Join the People's Medical Society.

The People's Medical Society *Newsletter* and our many other publications offer you an easy-to-read supply of medical information that you can use to make informed decisions about your health care.

135.
Plan a fire escape route, and hold home fire drills.

Simple fire-safety measures such as smoke alarms – an ample number placed strategically in your home – and fire drills can prevent serious injury or worse in the event of a home fire.

136.
Exercise regularly.

Regular exercise protects against heart disease, osteoporosis, and a variety of other common illnesses. It will also help you maintain a desirable weight. Joining a health club is cheaper than health care for a chronic illness such as heart disease.

137.
Make friends, and purchase a pet.

Studies have shown that people who are socially active are healthier than those who are "loners." Check your local newspaper for singles activities at churches, social organizations, Parents Without Partners, exercise clubs, and so on. Place an ad in the personals section of newspapers and magazines, or be daring and answer one!

Pets make great companions, and there are many dogs and cats at your local animal shelter just waiting for adoption. You'll have a lifelong friend and the satisfaction that comes with helping a less fortunate creature. How you feel mentally has long been connected to how you feel physically, and being socially active or having a pet are two ways to improve your health. And remember, the cost for dog and cat food is considerably less than the cost of multiple doctor visits and prescription medications.

138.
Wear a lead apron for dental X rays.

You should always shield the parts of your body not being X-rayed. Excessive radiation is a definite health hazard—and why invite trouble (and additional costs) when there's a simple remedy?

139.
Keep current with immunizations.

Adults need to be reimmunized periodically for tetanus and, in some areas of the country, other diseases as well. These immunizations often are given free or at a very low cost through community groups. Elderly adults, in particular, should consider immunization against influenza and pneumonia.

140.
Avoid too much exposure to the sun.

Dermatologists have definitely identified a link between exposure to the sun and skin cancer; however, you don't have to live in a cave. Some commonsense approaches to the sun are: Always use a sunscreen with a sun protection factor (SPF) of 15 or more; keep your exposure to a minimum; don't get all your sun at once; and wear protective clothing such as a hat or long-sleeved shirt when in the sun.

For more information on how to enjoy the sun and avoid the hazards, contact:

Skin Cancer Foundation
475 Park Avenue
New York, NY 10016

141.
Wash your hands.

Frequent hand washing will lower your chances of catching colds, flu, and other contagious diseases.

142.
Take a vacation.

Everyone needs and benefits from periodic breaks in the daily routine. Listen to yourself–don't get too "burned out" before you give yourself a break. Hotels are cheaper than hospitals.

143.
Get enough sleep.

Most people need seven to eight hours of sleep per day. Again, listen to yourself and make sure you get what you need.

144.
Eat lots of fiber.

Increasing the amount of fiber in your diet is the easiest way to lower your risk of colon cancer. It will also help with constipation. Laxatives are much more expensive than an extra piece of whole wheat bread.

145.
Drink cranberry juice.

Cranberry juice can be protective against bladder infections. But be careful to avoid the juices with added sugar and corn syrups. Cranberry juice is cheaper than antibiotics–and a lot more fun to ingest.

146.
Brush your teeth and floss daily.

Good oral hygiene is essential to good general health, so don't forget to brush and floss your teeth on a daily basis. Failure to develop and practice good oral health habits can be counter-productive to all your efforts at staying healthy. In addition, one unforeseen dental bill can wipe out any savings you've accumulated by practicing good general health.

Buy a plaque removal system for you and your family. Gum disease is one of the leading causes of tooth loss, and the cost to replace lost teeth can be quite high.

147.
Contact a self-help support group.

For many illnesses, a self-help support group can be as helpful as your doctor in speeding your recovery. Self-help support groups are in the business of empowerment, giving consumers the information and strategies they need to successfully deal with their conditions. In addition, in such groups you meet people who share your condition and with whom you can share a common bond. For more information on self-help groups, contact:

American Self-Help Clearinghouse
St. Clares-Riverside Medical Center
Denville, NJ 07834
201-625-7101

National Self-Help Clearinghouse
City University of New York
Graduate Center, Room 620
25 West 43rd Street
New York, NY 10036
212-642-2944

148.
Practice safe sex.

Unfortunately and undeniably, sexually transmitted diseases—
gonorrhea, herpes, syphilis, acquired immunodeficiency syndrome
(AIDS), just to name a few—are a nasty fact of life. Most at risk
are those people who have many sexual partners. The risks, however, are minimized if a condom is always used during intercourse.

149.
Know the number for your local poison control center.

Calling for help immediately if you suspect someone in your
family has ingested a poisonous substance can make the difference
between a minor digestive disturbance and a week in the hospital's
intensive care unit. Prompt action saves lives and money.

150.
Wear appropriate protective clothing when playing sports or engaging in recreational activities.

Whether the activity is bicycling or football, protective clothing
can spare participants from easily preventable injuries. Preventing
injuries or lessening their severity saves money.

Adverse reaction: Reaction that harms a person in some way.

Advocate: Person who represents another's interests.

Antihistamine: Medication used to treat allergies and cold symptoms such as itchy eyes and a runny nose.

Assignment: Process by which a doctor or hospital agrees to file an insurance claim in exchange for direct payment from the insurer. Under the Medicare system, the physician or hospital must also agree to accept that direct payment, plus any required patient copayments, as payment in full.

Audiologist: Medical practitioner (non-M.D.) who specializes in treating hearing problems.

Board certification: Medical specialty boards, such as the American College of Obstetricians and Gynecologists and the American Academy of Family Physicians, certify physicians in their respective specialties through a process of testing and evaluating qualifications.

Cesarean section: Method of delivering a baby by abdominal surgery.

Chiropractor: Medical practitioner (D.C.) who focuses on improving nerve function through manipulation and adjustment of body parts, particularly the spine.

Consultation: Discussion between physicians about a medical case or its treatment, for which the patient is billed.

Contraindication: Something that makes a particular medication or treatment inadvisable.

Copayment: Payment required of the patient in addition to the payment made by the insurance company. A copayment may be in the form of a deductible or a percentage payment (for instance, the insurance company pays 80 percent and the patient pays 20 percent).

Custodial care: Provision of room, board, and personal services, generally on a long-term basis, without additional medical services.

Decongestant: Medication that acts to clear congestion. It helps such symptoms as stuffy nose or chest congestion.

Deductible: Amount a patient is required to pay before his or her insurance company will begin to make payments.

Diagnosis: Identification of a patient's illness through consideration of the signs and symptoms.

Drug: Substance other than food that is intended to influence the functions of the body.

Family practitioner: Medical practitioner who specializes in treating the whole family, from uncomplicated births to care of the elderly.

For-profit: A business that operates to make more money than it requires to continue operating.

Generic drug: Drug that is a copy of a brand name drug.

Group insurance coverage: Insurance policy that covers a group of people. Such insurance is generally cheaper than individual coverage because the insurance risks are spread out among the group.

Health maintenance organization (HMO): Organization of medical providers that contracts with patients to offer specific services in exchange for a prepaid premium.

Hospice: Organization that provides specialized care for dying patients either in their home or at a facility.

Intermediate care facility: Facility that provides less intensive care than a skilled nursing facility. Patients are generally more mobile, and rehabilitation therapies are stressed.

Invasive treatment: Medical treatment that involves the invasion of the body with a drug or an instrument.

Itemized bill: Bill that lists each item and service and its corresponding charge.

Living will: Document that indicates a person's treatment wishes in the event that he or she is unable to verbally communicate those wishes. A living will is usually used as written authorization for the non-use or removal of life-sustaining treatments.

Midwife: Medical practitioner, often a nurse, who specializes in caring for women and delivering babies.

Nonprofit: Organization that functions by earning just enough money to continue operating.

Nosocomial infection: Infection acquired in the hospital.

Nurse practitioner: Nurse who has received specialized training that enables him or her to provide basic diagnostic medical care to patients.

Optometrist: Medical practitioner (O.D.) who specializes in examining eyes and who is able to prescribe corrective lenses but not perform surgery or invasive treatments.

Over-the-counter (OTC) drug: Drug that is available without a doctor's prescription.

Physician's assistant: Medical practitioner who is specially trained to provide a basic level of diagnostic medical care, usually under the supervision of a physician.

Physician's Desk Reference (PDR): A comprehensive reference book primarily listing prescription drugs and indications for use, contraindications, and dosages.

Podiatrist: Medical practitioner (D.P.M.) who specializes in caring for feet.

Preferred provider organization (PPO): Similar to an HMO, an organization of health care providers that contracts with patients for a specific amount of service in exchange for a prepaid premium.

Prescription drug: Drug that can be purchased only with a doctor's prescription.

Second opinion: An objective evaluation, diagnosis, and treatment recommendation from a medical practitioner concerning a health problem that has previously been evaluated by another medical practitioner.

Side effect: Effect of a drug or treatment that is not directly a part of the healing process.

Skilled nursing facility (SNF): An institution that offers nursing services similar to those given in a hospital, to aid recuperation of those who are seriously ill.